Masks, Misinformation, and Making Do

# Masks, Misinformation, and Making Do

## Appalachian Health-Care Workers and the COVID-19 Pandemic

Edited by Wendy Welch

Foreword by Alan Morgan

OHIO UNIVERSITY PRESS

ATHENS

Ohio University Press, Athens, Ohio 45701
ohioswallow.com
© 2023 by Ohio University Press

Printed in the United States of America
Ohio University Press books are printed on acid-free paper ∞ ™

Library of Congress Cataloging-in-Publication Data
Names: Welch, Wendy, editor. | Morgan, Alan (Of National Rural Health
    Association), writer of foreword.
Title: Masks, misinformation, and making do : Appalachian health-care
    workers and the COVID-19 pandemic / edited by Wendy Welch ; foreword
    by Alan Morgan.
Description: Athens : Ohio University Press, [2023] | Includes bibliographical
    references and index.
Identifiers: LCCN 2022036108 (print) | LCCN 2022036109 (ebook) | ISBN
    9780821425022 (paperback ; alk. paper) | ISBN 9780821425015 (hardcover ;
    alk. paper) | ISBN 9780821447864 (pdf)
Subjects: MESH: COVID-19—epidemiology | Rural Health Services | Health
    Personnel—psychology | Burnout, Professional | Health Services Accessi-
    bility | Social Determinants of Health | Appalachian Region—epidemiology
Classification: LCC RA644.C67 (print) | LCC RA644.C67 (ebook) | NLM
    WC 506.4 AA6 | DDC 362.1962/41440097568—dc23/eng/20220914
LC record available at https://lccn.loc.gov/2022036108
LC ebook record available at https://lccn.loc.gov/2022036109

*Death leaves a heartache no one can heal,*
*love leaves a memory no one can steal.*

—from an Irish headstone

*If you lost someone beloved during COVID,*

*this book is dedicated to you.*

# Contents

# Foreword

The emergence of the COVID-19 pandemic highlighted systemic shortcomings of our current health-care system and the subsequent impact of these shortcomings on the lives of underserved populations. However, the ongoing pandemic also provides us with an opportunity to test new models of care and to potentially, fundamentally, change the health-care landscape in the United States.

As chief executive officer of the National Rural Health Association, I have a unique perspective on this historic event, as both a national participant in and observer of the best and worst the pandemic has wrought upon our rural communities. This thoughtfully curated publication attempts to collect lessons learned and to provide first-hand success stories to build upon as we all move forward together. The health policy development process often takes years, if not decades, from problem identification to policy development until ultimately resulting in practice implementation. However, the COVID-19 pandemic acted as an accelerant to this process, transforming care and reshaping the health-care system in an unprecedented manner.

Health-care payment policies drive health-care practice. It is often noted that form follows function in health care. A good example of this is that national efforts to create an "efficient health-care system" have also created a nationwide system of care poorly positioned for pandemic surge capacity. Rural communities, long struggling with workforce shortages, find themselves now competing nationally for the recruitment and retention of key health-care staff at a level and magnitude not seen before. In fact, we are now entering a level of workforce disruption and shortage in the health-care field that is simply unsustainable for the future unless systemic changes are undertaken.

After two years of the pandemic, the impact on rural under-served communities is particularly clear. Rural America has an older, sicker, and poorer population, which now relies on a health-care infrastructure that was never designed for pandemic care. National surveys suggest that large percentages of rural populations are also less inclined to employ basic public health measures, such as mask wearing, in public venues. These national trends and characteristics of rural communities resulted in data showing 80 percent higher infection rates per population and mortality rates nearly double per population only a year into the pandemic.

While the tragic impact of the pandemic on underserved populations was both projected and feared at the beginning, two areas of early success offer a hope for the future. First, prompt and substantial federal and state financial support stabilized the health-care safety net. Second, punctual regulatory flexibility efforts removed barriers to innovation in the areas of telehealth and staffing. Thus, these two critical interventions by policy leaders at both the state and federal levels allowed innovation to flourish on many levels among health-care providers as the system adapted to the crisis at hand.

Therefore, the "story" of rural America during the COVID-19 pandemic is best examined by looking at the response of an under-resourced and poorly designed system of care, providing care for a population most at risk for the pandemic. In this backdrop, there exist stories of both innovation and success amidst the national tragedy.

Telehealth, in all forms and functions, certainly greatly ex-panded in usage and flourished as a necessity of the pandemic. Barriers to telehealth implementation, including licensure restric-tions, reimbursement for services rendered, both patient and cli-nician adoption, together allowed many communities to finally adopt new access avenues to care not previously available. In some cases, existing telehealth solutions, long adopted in a prepandemic environment, proved to be valuable resources in crisis situations as well. Project ECHO is one such example, a nationally recog-nized program adopted in many rural facilities as a synchronous provider-to-provider and peer-to-peer telemonitoring model that connects community providers with specialists. An examination of success stories such as Project ECHO can offer pathways to broader national implementation going forward.

Many rural facilities facing pandemic surges of care implemented new staffing patterns, which allowed health-care practitioners to practice at the top of their educational and licensure abilities. These models of staffing during the crisis periods offer a promising range of options to address long-standing health-care workforce problems.

In many rural underserved communities, the pandemic has further driven health care outside the walls of the local hospital. Schools, public health departments, oral health-care providers, behavioral health professionals, and others all play a vital role in community health. The pandemic-induced collaboration and networking that occurred across provider type and health-care settings have provided models of improved community health that can be applied in the future.

Perhaps among the greatest takeaways of the pandemic to date are the lessons learned on what it truly means to be a rural access point of care. Stories of success raise important policy questions regarding necessary capacity and services down the road. In particular, if rural hospitals are to remain focused solely on delivery of primary care and general surgery, then what networks of care and formal patient transfer arrangements are necessary for the future?

The final endpoint of the COVID-19 pandemic remains elusive. Rural health-care providers continue to see waves of infections among communities that have grown weary of the public health measures. Workforce challenges persist that only seem to grow more challenging with the passing of time. In the midst of these most challenging times, now is a prudent time to take stock of success stories and identify strategies, programs, and processes that can be replicated as we continue to navigate these most unprecedented times.

—*Alan Morgan, CEO, National Rural Health Association*

# Preface

Recently I listened to a prepandemic lecture talking about health-care heroism. The speaker said it was easy to find heroes in a crisis, but the real test of character was whether someone could be a friend through thick and thin, not to mention over very long hauls. Friends try to keep us from getting sick in the first place, stay with us when we are, and hold our hands as we make a journey to either recovery or the end of our lives.

Enthusiasm for "Heroes Work Here" signs outside hospitals waxed and waned as the pandemic's infectious waves rose and fell. We are all tired, none more so than those who went from heroes to scapegoats in public opinion. So I say the people who write of their experiences in this book, who share their expertise to explain what happened before and during the pandemic—not to mention what will likely come after—are not heroes, but something even more valuable and enduring. They are friends of humanity.

—*Wendy Welch*

# Acknowledgments

Books are never accomplished within a vacuum seal of writers. Many thanks are due to the board members of the Graduate Medical Education Consortium (GMEC) spanning the two years of this work. Also thanks to the residency program directors in GMEC's service area and beyond, who gave up "time off" to offer thoughts during one of the most stressful eras in the history of medicine. Thanks in particular to Lyn O'Connell for connecting us to West Virginia and Pennsylvania voices and to Melissa Zook and Chris Green for connections in Kentucky.

Many thanks go to photographer Elissa Powers, who first suggested the artist for the cover now gracing this volume. I would like to express my undying gratitude to M. J. Hiblen for his gracious gift of the cover art, which so beautifully captures the spirit of those fighting the virus.

It is a truth universally acknowledged that being married to a writer is a difficult gig, for many reasons. Jack Beck, husband par excellence, kept the home fires burning and the volume editor fed without editorial comment.

The nurses who got vaccinated, convinced others to vaccinate, endured gaslighting, made personal decisions about who to work for and why, and still showed up every day to hold the hands of frightened people who mistrusted them and everything else at the hospital cannot be adequately thanked. Words will never be enough for what you have endured or what you have offered during these pandemic years. You have been and will be on the right side of history.

# Part 1

## BACKGROUND

# 1

## Rural Medicine Retrospective

*An Overview of the Challenges Rural Hospitals Faced Prepandemic*

BETH O'CONNOR

*Editor's Note: Appalachia encompasses urban and rural areas, which suffered differently in the early pandemic stages. Where urban regions had swift and significant infection rates and loss of life, rural areas lost lives and future capacity in nuanced patterns that rarely garnered policy or media attention. To understand what happened in rural hospitals across America requires a little backgrounding. Challenges encumbered rural hospitals before the pandemic and exacerbated many of them. How will these troubles affect postpandemic medicine delivery?*

### THE HILL-BURTON ACT

As of April 1, 1945, nearly 5,000,000 male registrants between the ages of 18 and 37 had been examined and classified as unfit for military service. The number of those rejected for military service was about 30 percent of all those examined.

> —President Harry S. Truman, Special Message to the
> Congress Recommending a Comprehensive Health Program[1]

In the aftermath of World War II, Americans were shocked to realize how many men (and women) were unable to serve because of underlying health conditions. President Truman was determined to assure that every American had access to adequate health care in the future and proposed a five-point plan:

1. Increase the number of health-care professionals in low-income and rural communities

2. Create a robust public health system

3. Invest in medical research and medical education

4. Control the cost of receiving health care

5. Assure that a serious illness did not also cut off income

Results for the first item came quickly. The Hospital Survey and Construction Act (commonly referred to as the Hill-Burton Act for the senators who sponsored it) was signed into law in 1946. Federal grants and guaranteed loans were given to states and then passed down for communities to build new hospitals and modernize existing ones.

The goal was to provide 4.5 hospital beds for every 1,000 people. For modern-day Lee County, Virginia, that would mean at least 105 hospital beds for their current population of 23,500. Mercer County, West Virginia, should have 480 beds for their population of 107,300.

In 24 years, Hill-Burton funds supported the construction of 10,748 projects. An amount of $3.7 billion in federal funding was matched with an additional $9.1 billion from state and local governments and nonprofit organizations. Nearly a half million beds were created in hospitals and nursing homes, along with specialty facilities and public health centers. Adjusted for inflation, the combined $12.8 billion would equal over $81 billion taxpayer dollars in 2020.

For many years, the hospitals thrived, and their communities thrived with them. Community-based hospitals supported the growth of related industries such as food service, medical labs, and specialty care. A growing postwar economy, combined with an increased emphasis on workplace safety, created the need for occupational health services in every community. The baby boom required maternity wards and obstetricians. Rural hospitals became an economic driver everywhere they were located. The National Center for Rural Health Works estimates that a "rural primary care physician practicing in a community with a local hospital creates an estimated 26.3 local jobs and nearly $1.4 million in income (wages, salaries and benefits) from the clinic and the hospital."[2]

### PPS, EMTALA, AND THE CREATION OF CRITICAL ACCESS HOSPITALS

> Twenty-one percent of the U.S. population lives in rural areas. However, rural physicians comprise only about 10 percent of the total number of working physicians in the country.
>
> —American Academy of Family Physicians[3]

In an effort to decrease the burden on American taxpayers, the Centers for Medicaid and Medicare Services created a fixed price structure for all procedures, regardless of the actual cost. Starting in 1983, with various exceptions, the price was the price, whether the facility was located in New York City or Clintwood, Virginia, population 1,304.

While the assumption might be that costs would be higher in urban areas than rural, the reverse is often true in health care because of the efficiency that comes with volume. An urban hospital that does five intubations a day has a lower cost per procedure than a rural facility that performs the technique five times a week, much less five times a month. Additionally, a rural hospital will have a higher percentage of patients on Medicare and Medicaid, while the urban facility will have a higher percentage on private insurance to which the hospital can charge more than the actual cost to offset the loss from publicly funded patients.

The new price structure was dubbed the Prospective Payment System (PPS) and dictated that Medicare payments be made based on a predetermined, fixed amount. PPS created a complex classification system for each type of diagnosis in each setting that left little room for interpretation on a case-by-case basis.

Three years later, Congress passed the Emergency Medical Treatment and Active Labor Act (EMTALA), and any hospital covered under Medicare's PPS was now also subject to EMTALA. Prior to this, some hospitals had engaged in "patient dumping." Patients arrived at a hospital emergency department only to be turned away because of citizenship status or lack of ability to pay. Ambulances would commonly bypass a for-profit hospital and drive much farther to a nonprofit or public hospital, risking the patient's life with the extra time. Hospital executives labeled patients without insurance as GOOMERS—Get Out of My Emergency Room.

EMTALA required that any patient in an emergency department be screened and stabilized prior to transferring the patient to a different facility, but the mandate was unfunded. Hospitals could bill the patient for services received, yet there was no guarantee of payment. Nationwide, approximately 6 percent of hospital visits are not covered by insurance. In rural America that number is much higher, with 10 to 15 percent of rural patients unable to foot the bill themselves.[4]

Indirectly, EMTALA also led to people without insurance visiting the emergency department for nonemergencies. They knew that they would not be turned away without at least a basic screening, and thus emergency departments became the primary care provider for many. Between 1993 and 2003, emergency department visits grew by 26 percent.[5]

The result of PPS and EMTALA was hospital closures: 440 rural hospitals closed between 1985 and 1992.[6] Rural health advocates eventually gained the attention of Congress regarding the unintended consequences of the regulations. A series of policy initiatives were passed to benefit rural facilities, including State Offices of Rural Health, Medicare Dependent Hospitals, the Medicare Rural Flexibility Program, Low-Volume Hospital Adjustment, and Critical Access Hospitals. Together, these programs were designed to stabilize the rural health-care safety net.

The Critical Access Hospital (CAH) designation provided vulnerable rural facilities with benefits to assure that essential services remained available in rural communities. The most notable benefit became cost-based reimbursement. Instead of having to stick to the Medicare PPS payment caps, CAH facilities are allowed to submit for the actual cost of a procedure, plus an additional 1 percent. A few states took this policy a step further and approved 101 percent reimbursement for Medicaid claims as well.

The eligibility for designation as a CAH is very strict:

- Have 25 or fewer acute care inpatient beds
- Be located more than 35 miles from another hospital (some exceptions made for mountainous terrain and other special situations)
- Maintain an annual average length of stay of 96 hours or less for acute care patients
- Provide 24/7 emergency care services

Nearly 1,400 hospitals in the nation achieved CAH status.[7] Other rural hospitals received financial support through the Medicare Dependent Hospitals program, Medicaid disproportionate share hospital payments, or the Low-Volume Hospital Adjustment. While not every rural entity was able to participate, the new policies were a lifeline to many rural hospitals. Providers previously on the brink of closure stabilized and even thrived in some places.

THE LOSS OF INDEPENDENT COMMUNITY HOSPITALS

Hospital mergers and acquisitions are changing the face of health care in both rural and urban communities across the country. For many rural hospitals, the financial choice may be to merge or go out of business.

—North Carolina Rural Health Research Program[8]

By 2005, the earliest Hill-Burton facilities were approaching 60 years old. Many of them had infrastructure that was outdated or worse, and many of the nonprofits, small towns, and counties that had founded the hospitals wanted to get out of the health-care business.

There were major reasons to look elsewhere for hospital management. Medicare cost controls required updated technology and other improvements that were beyond the capacity of a small, standalone facility. Regional health-care systems were more cost-effective by consolidating services into a single location rather than maintaining and staffing multiple small volume sites. And finally, a high percentage of patients not covered by higher-paying private insurance combined with a low patient volume meant that many rural facilities were unsustainable.

Between 2005 and 2016, small communities saw their locally controlled hospital snapped up by urban-based health-care systems; 380 hospital mergers took place nationwide.[8] Some systems bought out other systems, which meant that rural citizens observed the signs in front of their facility change more than once.

Health-care systems viewed the acquisition of rural hospitals (and clinics) as a way to expand their referral system; a patient with needs beyond the expertise of the primary care providers is directed to specialists. The creation of regional health-care systems meant that specialty services for insured patients would not take place at the rural facility. Before merger, a physician at an unaffiliated clinic could send a patient to the specialist that the physician or patient preferred. A specialist could be chosen due to proximity to the patient, experience with the particular symptoms, or any other reason.

After the merger, there would be strong pressure to keep the patient within the health-care system. Unless it was an emergency (and often, even if it was), that heart catheterization would not take place in a rural community. A patient arriving at a CAH facility would be stabilized, then loaded into an ambulance (ground or air) and transported to the main facility that dominated the region. Where the patient went, their private insurance payment followed and went to the system hub facility, while responsibility for paying the ambulance ($40,000 or more for air transport) was stuck on the patient.

In nonemergency situations, in-system referrals mean that the patient sometimes had to travel past a specialist in a nearby community to get to the preferred provider. Referral pathways proved an effective way of keeping patients with good insurance from going to the competition for health care.

Hospital mergers meant loss of services and loss of control in the local community. Many services, such as orthopedic surgery, were no longer available in hometowns as consolidation into a single system-wide location absorbed the specialists. Maternity wards closed. Doctors, nurses, and other hospital staff were no longer employed by the local facility, but by the urban umbrella, or even by a third-party staffing contractor. Along with the services and the staff, the tax revenue previously generated by local hospital employees and services shifted toward the city, further damaging rural economies.

Rural employers felt the pinch of hospital mergers indirectly. Preemployment screenings were now subject to decisions made outside of the job site. The ability to negotiate rates with health insurance providers became severely restricted when there was only one health-care system for the insurance company to consider.

In some cases, hospital mergers meant that a health-care system made big promises to a local community that it was not able to keep. In ten instances, the urban system purchased the local facility and then closed the doors within five years. Community members felt duped and wondered aloud: Did the system purchase the hospital just to strip it of valuable equipment?

## THE RISE OF TELEHEALTH

> By removing barriers of time, distance, and provider scarcities,
> telehealth can deliver important medical and other health and
> education services where they are needed most; in remote,
> rural areas and medically underserved urban communities.
>
> —Mid-Atlantic Telehealth Resource Center[9]

A consistent issue in rural health care is the lack of specialists in rural communities. Hospital mergers provided a partial solution for those under the umbrella, but independent clinics and the hospitals that were unaffiliated still could not provide access services outside of primary care without significant expense to their patients. While the ratio of specialists to population in urban areas is 263 per 100,000, rural communities have only 30 per 100,000.[8] Rural communities have been consistently unable to recruit or retain psychiatrists, orthopedic surgeons, pain management specialists, or any of the host of people with a job title ending in "-ologist."

As the ability of the internet grew, telehealth was proposed as a viable alternative to in-person specialty visits. A specialist in another town or even another state than the patient could evaluate anything viewable on a computer screen. Blood pressure, CT scan, ultrasound, cardiogram, and the actual patient could be checked remotely.

Just like the hospital mergers, telehealth came with its own set of benefits and concerns. There is no need to have an obstetrician in a small town when a fetal monitor can be reviewed 500 miles away. Why pay for a physician in your intensive care unit when it can be staffed with nurse practitioners who have virtual access to an intensive care unit specialist with the ability to monitor several hospitals at once? Many facilities were so excited that they could provide services virtually that they did not stop to consider what the unintended consequences would be, while opportunists saw telehealth as a new way to make money. Moving services online continued the trend of decreasing the physical presence of health-care professionals in rural communities and rural economies.

THE AFFORDABLE CARE ACT AND MEDICAID (NON) EXPANSION

139 Rural Hospitals have closed since 2010.

—Cecil G. Sheps Center for Health Services Research[10]

In 2010, Congress passed the Patient Protection and Affordable Care Act (ACA), and it was quickly signed into law by President Obama, who had made increased access to health care a cornerstone of his campaign. Praised by some as "the Affordable Care Act" and derided by others as "O-bummer-care," the ACA included something that hospitals lobbied hard to receive: the individual mandate.

Prior to the ACA, no one was required to have health insurance, but EMTALA still required hospitals to treat anyone who showed up in the emergency department. Patients without an ability to pay were a burden for all hospitals, but more so for rural facilities with a higher percentage of self-employed farmers, small business owners without traditional insurance, and others lacking a way to pay. The 10 to 15 percent uninsured made it difficult for many rural facilities to keep their doors open, even with the adjustments to the Medicare payments. It does not take much to imagine what would happen to a grocery, clothing store, or apartment complex if 15 percent of customers did not pay their bills.

Hospitals were so eager to have a requirement that everyone be insured that they agreed to a lower Medicare rate. Less money from Medicare was a good trade if more patients could at least pay something; but not everyone supported the idea that purchasing insurance should be a requirement of US citizens.

In 2012, the Affordable Care Act was challenged in the Supreme Court. Many hoped that the individual mandate would be declared unconstitutional and struck down. Supporters of the requirement cheered when it was ruled that the individual mandate was acceptable. They cheered so loudly that the section of the ACA the Supreme Court ruled as unconstitutional was initially overlooked.

In order to decrease the number of people without insurance, the ACA proposed a massive expansion of state Medicaid programs. Prior to the ACA, states were only required to provide Medicaid to those with disabilities that prevented them from working, pregnant women, and mothers of small children. People who simply did not make enough money to buy health insurance did not qualify for Medicaid in many states.

The ACA provided funding for states to increase eligibility for Medicaid. People who worked in low-income jobs who previously could not afford private insurance would qualify for the Medicaid program under ACA. What the Supreme Court ruled was that the federal government had no authority to force states to accept the funds and expand Medicaid.

Political pandemonium followed. A few states immediately accepted the expansion funds and put the expanded Medicaid programs into place. Many states accepted Medicaid expansion only after years of partisan wars. Some states still refuse expansion funds.

For rural hospitals, refusing expansion pulled the life support plug. The Supreme Court decision meant that they still had uninsured patients in their emergency department, but they also had the lower Medicare payments that were part of the ACA negotiations. The deal had been broken on both ends.

The fallout was immediate. Within months, hospitals that had been on the edge of survival closed their doors, leaving communities without access to emergency services. To date, 139 rural hospitals have closed and another 450 are considered vulnerable. More than half of the affected communities saw any clinic or satellite service affiliated with the hospital closed as well. Some 60 percent of the closed hospitals are in the South. Almost all of them are in states that refused to expand Medicaid.

DEATH BY A THOUSAND CUTS—THE RURAL HOSPITAL CRISIS

The rate of closure has steadily increased since sequestration began and bad debt cuts began to hit rural hospitals, resulting in a rate six times higher in 2015 compared to 2010.

—National Rural Health Association[10]

Lack of Medicaid expansion was only the beginning. Political fights combined with a desire to reduce the burden on American taxpayers meant that Congress made additional reductions in Medicaid payments to hospitals; nothing big: 1 percent here, 2 percent there, not big enough to catch the attention of lawmakers unfamiliar with the need to support rural facilities or the thin financial line that divided open from closed.

In addition to the payment cuts, pressure grew for hospitals to bear the responsibility for the overall health of the people that lived in their service area. Referred to as "Population Health Management," hospitals now had to address public health issues such as obesity and substance misuse or risk losing even more money. And they had to do it whether the individuals living in the local community wanted help or not.

Talking heads often stereotype rural communities as "older, poorer, sicker." Like many sound bites, this perspective is both harmful and true. Providing care in a community where one-fifth of your population is over age 65, the average income is 20 percent lower than the national average, and people are likely to have six or more chronic conditions is no easy task. Reducing those chronic conditions without significant resources proves nearly impossible. Hospital leaders started using the phrase "patient responsibility" to voice their frustration over the inability to control individual choices to eat healthy, exercise more, and stop inappropriate substance use.

Nineteen rural hospitals closed in 2019 because of these challenges—the highest annual total since 2004. Research indicates that this number will not decrease in the years ahead.

### PREPARING FOR THE EMERGENCY

It isn't the number of cases that matter. It doesn't matter if you only have five cases. What matters is that you have five cases, but only three ICU beds.

—Ryan Kelly, Mississippi Rural Health Association[11]

In the wake of post-9/11 concerns about bioterrorism, all hospitals were required to update their Emergency Preparedness Plans to include infectious epidemics. Checklists were created, plans filed, and mock drills instigated. But the plans could only do so much in a rural hospital infrastructure designed to push every patient it could to an affiliated urban center.

Enter COVID-19. Dealing with a pandemic requires both financial resources and human capital. In a rush to try to keep COVID-19 out of the United States, the White House administration placed a ban on foreign visas. This good intention had the result of cutting off the supply of health-care providers from other countries and sending home many of those already practicing in the United States. International medical graduates receive visas that allow them to practice in rural and underserved urban areas, which provides a path to permanent residency. Foreign doctors are one-quarter of the total physician workforce in the United States. A ban on foreign visas meant a reduction of 15,000 physicians in rural and inner-city communities.[12] In response to a health-care crisis, rural America had fewer doctors than before.

Tiny operating margins mean that most rural hospitals and clinics have very little reserves in terms of funds, supplies, or staffing. The initial response to COVID-19 meant that most facilities ceased all nonemergency procedures in order to avoid spreading infection. In rural communities, that meant that the few procedures that could still be done on-site ceased.

No procedures meant no incoming payments from insurance companies. No payments meant layoff for health-care providers who did not staff the emergency departments or intensive care units at a time when operations should be ramping up to prepare for the wave of COVID infections. Revenue disappeared.

No cash reserves meant no supply reserves. Rural facilities do not have a warehouse of masks, gloves, shoe covers, or test swabs. The tiny supply closet runs out quickly when orders must be small and frequent. A run on the precious N95 respirators in major metropolitan areas left none available for rural sites. Even the systems created by hospital mergers did not have the buying power of urban institutions. A group of clinics in rural Virginia got the idea to band together to submit a large order in the hopes of being able to receive them quickly. The N95 respirators showed up two months later; hand sanitizer did not arrive for three months.

Outside of health care, rural economic drivers increased the spread of COVID-19. When you say "rural," urban people tend to picture a lone farmer on a tractor in the middle of a field, generating a sense of low risk in pandemic conditions. However, independent farmers have given way to factory farms and meatpacking plants. With a high dependency on immigrants working long hours in close quarters, many rural communities went from zero cases to being a hot spot almost overnight. Infection rates in communities with meatpacking plants were five times higher than the rest of rural America.[13]

State and federal prisons are mostly located in rural America. From 2013 to 2019, prison populations shot up 27 percent in rural areas.[14] Overcrowding can mean less programming, fewer services, unsafe conditions, and more time locked down in cells. This can lead jails that already struggle with limited resources and infrastructure to become further plagued with abuse, poor health care, and abysmal conditions. Inmates packed into an overcrowded building meant that 80 percent of the prisoners, along with 160 employees at a correctional institution in rural Ohio, were infected.[15] As of mid-December 2020, one in every five prisoners in the United States had tested positive for the coronavirus, a rate more than four times as high as the general population.[16]

And where did urbanites with means go to get away from it all? They went to rural America. When social distancing guidelines were first released, wealthy urban Americans packed up their families and headed to vacation homes and resorts in rural communities. This wasn't unique to Appalachia. The influx of people from outside overwhelmed local capacity across rural America when city citizens brought COVID-19 along with their suitcases. Ski resort communities in Colorado, Utah, and Idaho were hard hit, with Idaho's Wood River Valley spiking at 192 cases and two deaths in a county of only 22,000 people.[17] The hospital in Twin Falls, Idaho, was overrun and unable to transfer patients to Boise because hospitals there were also over capacity.

Another complication in a rural response to a pandemic is the culture of rural communities. People like to throw around the phrase "tight-knit" to describe the interconnectedness in small towns. Treating the patient in Exam Room 3 takes on a whole new meaning when that person is also your aunt—or your neighbor, or your choir director, or your high school principal. Here's the fun part: that patient in Exam Room 3 could easily be your aunt and your neighbor and your choir director and your high school principal—all at once. Many health-care providers joke about the impossibility of following the Health Insurance Portability and Accountability Act (HIPAA) guidelines in rural communities. Social distancing in such situations is beyond belief.

Hospital mergers combined with telehealth had stripped necessary services from local communities. The Kaiser Family Foundation reported that more than half of US counties are without any ICU beds; an analysis completed by the Chartis Center for Rural

Health found that 63 percent of the nation's rural hospitals were without any ICU beds.

Most serious were the communities without any facilities at all. Remember that the Hill-Burton Act meant that Lee County, Virginia, should have 105 hospital beds and 480 beds in Mercer County, West Virginia? For some time, they had none; Lee County closed in 2010 after Virginia initially refused to expand Medicaid and then reopened in 2021 under different management, with a maximum capacity of 10 beds. Mercer County's Bluefield Regional Medical Center closed in July of 2020. Residents of those communities with health concerns had to go elsewhere.

### THE STORM

> The obstacles faced by health care providers and patients
> in rural areas are vastly different than those in urban areas.
> Economic factors, cultural and social differences, educa-
> tional shortcomings, lack of recognition by legislators and
> the sheer isolation of living in remote areas all conspire to
> create health care disparities and impede rural Americans in
> their struggle to lead normal, healthy lives.
>
> —National Rural Health Association[18]

Patchy insurance coverage, lack of providers, and shuttered rural hospitals combined to create a mighty health-care crisis. The *Daily Yonder,* an online newspaper for rural issues, reported that of the 100 counties nationally with the highest infection rates for May 2020, three-quarters were rural. By August, the weekly rate of new infections per 100,000 was 16.6 in rural counties versus 15.9 for the nation as a whole.[13]

President Truman communicated in 1945 a vision "that financial barriers in the way of attaining health shall be removed; that the health of all its citizens deserves the help of all the Nation."[1] He lost a vicious battle to establish a universal health-care system. It was attacked as "socialized medicine," with the Truman administration ridiculed as "followers of the Moscow party line." Truman later called the failure to pass a national health insurance program one of the most bitter and troubling disappointments in his presidency. He was on hand in 1965 when President Lyndon B. Johnson signed Medicare and Medicaid into law, with President Johnson proclaiming Truman as "the real daddy of Medicare."[19] It would be 45 more years before another step was taken forward, with the passage of the Affordable Care Act in 2010—a law that is also now in jeopardy.

Truman's vision of the nation was lost long before COVID-19 showed how lost it was. The cracks were there, and under pressure they opened into fissures of division and incapable systems that swallowed the lives of the marginalized, without comment or care as the whole world rushed to make up for lost time in righting these wrongs before the bill came due.

### REFERENCES

1 Truman, H. S. Special message to the Congress recommending a comprehensive health program. Harry S. Truman Library and Museum, November 19, 1945. https://www.trumanlibrary.gov/library /public-papers/192/special-message-congress-recommending -comprehensive-health-program.

2 Eilrich, F., Doeksen, G., St. Clair, C. Estimate the economic impact of a rural primary care physician. National Center for Rural Health Works, October 2016. https://ruralhealthworks.org/wp-content /uploads/2018/04/Physician-Impact-Study-Final-100416.pdf.

3 American Academy of Family Physicians. Rural practice, keeping physicians in. Position paper, 2014. https://www.aafp.org/about /policies/all/rural-practice-keeping-physicians.html.

4 Day, J.C. Rates of uninsured fall in rural counties, remain higher than urban counties. United States Census Bureau, April 9, 2019. https://www.census.gov/library/stories/2019/04/health-insurance -rural-america.html.

5 Centers for Disease Control and Prevention. Visits to U.S. emergency departments at all-time high; number of departments shrinking, last reviewed October 6, 2006. https://www.cdc.gov/nchs /pressroom/05news/emergencydept.htm.

6 Office of Inspector General, Department of Health and Human Services. Trends in rural hospital closure: 1987–1991. July 1993. https:// oig.hhs.gov/oei/reports/oei-04-92-00441.pdf.

7   Flex Monitoring Team. Critical access hospitals locations list. Last updated July 20, 2022. https://www.flexmonitoring.org/critical-access-hospital-locations-list.

8   Williams, D., Thomas, S., Howard, H., Pink, G. Rural hospital mergers from 2005 through 2016. North Carolina Rural Health Research Program, August 2018. https://www.shepscenter.unc.edu/wp-content/uploads/dlm_uploads/2018/08/Rural-Hospital-Mergers.pdf.

9   Mid-Atlantic Telehealth Resource Center. Why telehealth? https://www.matrc.org/what-is-telehealth/why-telehealth/. Accessed August 29, 2022.

10  Cecil G. Sheps Center for Health Services Research. Rural hospital closures. https://www.shepscenter.unc.edu/programs-projects/rural-health/rural-hospital-closures/. Accessed August 29, 2022.

11  Kelly, R. Facebook comment, 2020.

12  Pugh, T. Proposed visa renewal change carries doctor shortage risk. Bloomberg Law, October 19, 2020. https://news.bloomberglaw.com/health-law-and-business/proposed-visa-renewal-change-carries-doctor-shortage-risk?fbclid=IwAR0HJAHSk4oIV6G8X04ikZ7V8Q6DO7cX1BY-NiF1n1udZIlyVCDoiLgHcxo.

13  Covid-19 dashboard for rural America. *Daily Yonder,* 2020. https://dailyyonder.com/covid-19-dashboard-for-rural-america/.

14  Kang-Brown, J., Hinds, O., Schattner-Elmaleh, E., Wallace-Lee, J. People in jail in 2019. Vera, December 2019. https://www.vera.org/downloads/publications/people-in-jail-in-2019.pdf.

15  Bishop, B., Marema, T. Rural cases increase by a third over the last week. *Daily Yonder,* April 20, 2020. https://dailyyonder.com/rural-cases-increase-by-a-third-over-the-last-week/2020/04/20/.

16  Ollove, M. Analysis: How Covid-19 in prisons and jails threatens the surrounding community. *Daily Yonder,* July 2, 2020. https://dailyyonder.com/analysis-how-covid-19-in-prisons-and-jails-threatens-the-surrounding-community/2020/07/02/.

17  Carey, L. Covid, staffing shortages force Idaho hospitals to implement crisis standards of care. *Daily Yonder,* September 28, 2021. https://dailyyonder.com/covid-staffing-shortages-force-idaho-hospitals-to-implement-crisis-standards-of-care/2021/09/28/.

18  National Rural Health Association. About rural health care. https://www.ruralhealth.us/about-nrha/about-rural-health-care. Accessed August 29, 2022.

19  Markel, H. 69 years ago, a president pitches his idea for national health care. PBS News Hour, November 19, 2014. https://www.pbs.org/newshour/health/november-19-1945-harry-truman-calls-national-health-insurance-program.

# 2

---

# Good Hygiene in Bad Times

## ALLI DELP

*Editor's Note: The 1918 flu pandemic is often compared to the COVID-19 crisis, but several global illnesses reshaped human life throughout history. From a physician's perspective, these health crises also changed attitudes favorably toward population health initiatives and education. Here, a medical teaching faculty member explains what the virus does to bodies and, hopefully, its legacy on attitudes and home health practices regarding hygiene.*

P andemic, a world affected by a killer disease: Have we as a human species ever experienced anything like this before, and are we equipped to handle its effects? History says yes.

One of the earliest recorded pandemics is the Justinian plague that started in AD 541 and recurred over the next 200 years. It killed about 50 million people and prevented Emperor Justinian's plans to bring the Roman Empire back together. The Justinian plague is thought to be the first occurrence of the bubonic plague, but some historians believe accounts of bubonic plague were present in the Old Testament of the Bible, where accounts of Philistines who stole the Ark of the Covenant would succumb to "swellings."[1]

Next came the Black Death (200 million dead), which spanned from 1347 to 1351 and was caused by the bacterium *Yersinia pestis*, transmitted from parasites in fleas on rodents. It caused black sores on those infected, thus its name. Black Death can cause three different types of plague: bubonic (inflaming lymph nodes), pulmonic (respiratory), and septicemic (blood infection). Pulmonic and septicemic were usually fatal, but the bubonic plague had a 30–75 percent death rate.[2] Most of us know about this plague from history class because it caused massive death in a four-year time span and changed European society from the ground up. Among its sociological effects, people became more rebellious and questioned authority, demanding an end to serfdom.[2] Epidemic breakouts of this same plague continue in modern times, but modern medicine can now stop it in its tracks.

The last plague pandemic is considered to be the Third Plague (12 million dead), which was again due to the same flea-vectored bacterium, *Yersinia pestis*. This is the earliest that plague is recorded on the North and South American continents. The Third Plague led to the development of early public health measures to reduce infectious spreading. These prevention measures included hand hygiene, cleaning and disinfecting, and controlling the main distributor of the disease: rats.[1]

The last pandemic to mention was borne by parasites, but it was a different beast altogether. It was a virus. The infamous influenza pandemic of 1918–20 caused 17 million confirmed deaths, but the count could be as high as 100 million. It was caused by the H1N1 virus. At that time in history, a flu vaccine was not available to prevent infection. This flu was especially deadly to children under the age of 5, adults aged 20–40, and those 65 and older. It was unique in the fact that those aged 20–40, who were generally more healthy, had an extraordinarily high mortality rate.[3] Learning from this deadly flu outbreak helped the global public health community prepare for contemporary pandemics.[3]

One thing history shows is that there always will be another plague or pandemic on the horizon; combating these future threats requires learning from past outbreaks of illnesses. SARS-CoV-2, a.k.a. COVID-19, is no exception.

Health is generally a prominent concern in our society at political policy levels, but COVID-19 brought responses to a personal level. As a family practitioner in a rural community, I found myself explaining the differences between a virus and bacteria many times prepandemic. Patients would ask for antibiotics for viral infections, saying, "The last time I was sick like this I was given an antibiotic and I got better," or the ever-popular, "I don't have time to be sick right now; can't you just give me something to make this go away quickly?" Perhaps not much has changed from the time of the bubonic plagues in that regard.

Of course humans want quick fixes for ailments, but sometimes, as is the case with viral infections, none are available. Antibiotics don't work on viruses. Yet, given how much information and knowledge we have at our fingertips as a whole, we are still not as well educated as we should be about staying healthy—or perhaps just not compliant. Helping those outside the medical field to understand the importance of washing hands and vaccinations is difficult. People have head knowledge, but their actions do not follow their understanding. Among other things, the pandemic has been a terrible lesson in aerosol contagion and personal hygiene regarding washing hands and covering coughs. Perhaps by explaining in general terms what this novel coronavirus is, we can also inspire people to take steps to help combat it.

### WHAT IS A VIRUS?

A virus is a microscopic organism unable to reproduce on its own; it must be inside another living cell to replicate. It is made up of ribonucleic acid (RNA) or deoxyribonucleic acid (DNA). A virus is nonsentient yet alive, its acidic building blocks of life preprogrammed for two things: to survive and multiply. The moment a virus cell replicates, it begins seeking an optimal living environment where it can make more copies of itself. All humans and animals have DNA, and ours is pretty much programmed for that same baseline survival and replication. One quick clarification, though: DNA is double stranded, whereas RNA is single stranded; and RNA does not store genetic information, whereas DNA does.

A key factor to how well a virus survives is making sure that it does not kill its host before replicating multiple times. (High school teachers often use the movie *Aliens* to describe how viruses work: getting as much out of their host as they can before they use them up and move on; they are not wrong.) Viruses are difficult to treat because they mutate rapidly, and our immune system must continually create internal antibodies to these new mutations. This is part of the reason there is no cure or vaccine for the common cold. In fact, the reason we no longer die from most viruses is not so much medical intervention as the reality that those viruses have mutated to their advantage, making people only mildly ill in order to replicate and move on to the next host without killing the original host. Because if the original host dies, then the virus living in the host dies as well. In simple terms, it is in the best interests of any virus not to kill us.

Most viruses replicate only in certain host cells. Some viruses only infect plants, others only animals. Some viruses have such a narrow range of hosts that they can only infect primates (such as poliovirus). This means humans are not susceptible to every virus in the world. However, some viruses can mutate and combine with other viruses, enabling them to infect organisms they previously did not. This is a probable scenario that allowed humans to be susceptible to SARS-CoV-2. Bats are likely the primary source of this novel virus, but we do not know if COVID-19 is contracted directly from the bats or from other intermediate hosts.[4] The infection of a pangolin and then a human suggests the pandemic-causing coronavirus mutated to cross species and find better hosts from a viral point of view.

SARS-CoV-2, or COVID-19, is a coronavirus from the coronaviridae family, so named because they look like halos or crowns under a microscope. (You may remember the SARS virus scare [Avian Flu].) Although SARS-CoV-2 resembles the SARS virus, it is a novel mutation of a coronavirus. In other words, humans have not encountered the recently mutated virus before, and therefore have no immunity to it.

Viruses would be just plain fascinating, if they weren't so potentially deadly. One way a virus fights for its survival is mutation, to evade our immune system. Our system is gearing up to figure out what to attack, but meanwhile the enemy is changing into something our body doesn't recognize. Coronaviruses have a receptor-binding protein (RBP) on their spikes that initiates the invasion into a host cell. Studies found that coronaviruses have evolved to mask these RBPs from our body's antibody manufacturing system and to vary them among strains so that they will confuse the host immune system. This is the ultimate camouflage; such variations make it almost impossible for a host to recognize a new strain.[5] Hence, waiting for our bodies to figure out that the virus is camouflaged and replicating is not a good idea. Getting a vaccination of cells that do recognize the coronavirus protein spikes is a better idea; our body has antibodies before the virus hits and—in simple terms—doesn't have to start from scratch.

Typically, human bodies encounter a virus and find that it bears some resemblance to others sufficient to create antibodies. Then, when the body encounters that same virus again, the body can more quickly attack and get rid of the virus. Our bodies are wonderful creations that form immunities to invaders. This has, unfortunately, been used as a reason to avoid vaccination by some individuals. *Novel* and *virulent* are important words to remember when describing COVID-19. Even as your body attempts to mount a defense to an invader it has never seen before, you are getting sick. Your body is about to be very, very busy and quite possibly become overwhelmed in its defenses.

When SARS-CoV-2 enters our body, it floats around until it finds a cell to attack. Once attached to a cell via those famous protein spikes, the virus is able to get inside the host cell and create new viral particles. These particles will remain inside the cell undetected by our immune system until there are so many replicants that the cell ruptures and spills out all these virus particles. Think of a spider egg hatching; it is just about as creepy, honestly.

Thousands of particles are now inside the hapless human host, looking for cells to invade in order to make more and more virus particles. This continues until the virus has spread throughout its victim. Some areas of our insides are more welcoming to certain viruses, and it seems our lungs are particularly inviting to COVID-19.

Once this virus makes it into the lungs, it finds a moist, warm neighborhood suited to its needs and decides it is going to stay for a while. So it churns out more soldiers to protect its new cozy territory and goes to all-out war with our immune system. While in the lungs, it causes havoc, because as our body wages war against the virus, inflammation occurs. Our body produces cytokines, which are little messengers sent out to activate certain cells in our body to coordinate the effort to fight off the invader; COVID-19 creates an overwhelming cytokine storm. Inflammation is just a by-product of our immune system. The human host begins to get short of breath and will test positive for COVID.

TRANSMISSION

How did those viral organisms with the protein spikes get inside that human host in the first place? After a few months, the medical community learned that COVID-19 is aerosol spread (by inhalation of droplets and small airborne particles). A droplet that contains the coronavirus and its particles will enter our bodies either through our mouth, eyes, or nose. In addition to breathing it in, we can transmit it to other "points of entry" on our face via unwashed hands that have been exposed to droplets. From the moment that any virus finds its way inside us, it is up to our body to mount a response to the new invader.

In the simplest terms and ignoring complicating factors, breathing in an infected person's exhaled breath is the primary method of COVID-19 transmission. It took some time for airborne transmission to be solidified as the main form of transmission; remember the early advice to wipe down our groceries and mail? At first, COVID appeared to be easily transmitted airborne in short distances (less than 6 feet, hence the social distancing guidelines), but controversy developed over how far and how long the virus could travel; perfect lab conditions had it flying 27 feet, while other trials said 3 feet with mitigating factors like cold air and facing one another versus standing side by side. Early agreement was swift that it did not transmit via the fecal to oral route (like hepatitis A) or travel blood borne (like HIV).

A person infected with the virus is most contagious in the early stages of the illness—and would likely not be experiencing sufficient recognizable symptoms to tell them they are contagious. Physicians worldwide gave a collective groan of exasperation as this fact coalesced from experiences and observations combining into data showing a pattern. Risk of transmission also depends upon the type and duration of exposure to which one is subjected. Guidelines finally suggested that more than 10 minutes in close proximity to an infected person were necessary to contract the virus. Highest risks would come from someone living in the same household who brought the infection back to the home. Clusters of cases emerged after social or work gatherings where transmission occurred through close contact. And it was proven possible to contract the illness if one came in close contact while outdoors, even though the risk was much lower. Reduced risks outdoors sometimes translated to "no outdoor risk" in popular imagination, and that was patently untrue. The more masking (while in close quarters or indoors), ventilation, and social distance, the less risk one would have.

And, of course, the converse was true. The highest risks of transmission from exposure were quickly seen in congregate settings such as cruise ships, nursing homes, homeless shelters, and detention facilities.

Transmitting the illness from one person to another involves something called viral load, which is just what it sounds like. Those most contagious have the largest viral loads; the longer you are exposed to someone ill in a tight or unventilated space, the more viral load you are picking up. It is an intuitive concept similar to cigarette smoke exposure. If you stand near someone for two cigarettes, you may pick up the odor and will breathe in fumes.

That said, continued viral detection in respiratory swabs months after initial infection has been observed in many people previously infected with the virus.[4] Fortunately, a much higher viral load than what is found in those respiratory swabs would be needed to transmit infection to someone else; the RNA concentrations of the virus appear to be too low to cause infection, as noted by the Centers for

Disease Control and Prevention (CDC). In other words, at about the 3-day mark after recovery, with no symptoms or fever, a person who had COVID-19 has a very low chance of passing it to someone else. Transmission after 7–10 days of illness seems unlikely.[4] For months, a 10-day quarantine from the time of initial symptoms or positive test was considered standard to decrease spread of the virus, going down to 5 days as new information emerged (and as worker shortages began in many industries).

Indirect contact, such as passing an infected person on the street, touching an object that an infected individual coughed or sneezed on (and thus spread viral droplets onto), is now considered low risk. While initial research had us scrubbing down our groceries with scary declarations that the virus lived on certain surfaces up to 6 days, tested scenarios did not mimic actual conditions and this was eventually dropped from official recommendations.[6]

OUR BODIES AND SARS-COV-2

Say you did get infected; how would you know those infamous protein spikes were hard at work trying to break down your body's cells? In my clinic, we saw a spectrum of presentations, from asymptomatic to critical. A quick point of order here: some of those initially considered asymptomatic become symptomatic within 7 days, meaning they were actually presymptomatic. The main health concerns regarding asymptomatic patients is their probability to spread disease without knowing they are ill. Whether or not this is a main contributor to the spread of the illness will be debated in coming years within the medical community. Most patients presenting at my clinic with COVID symptoms and who subsequently tested positive had a known exposure to someone that was ill or presymptomatic. Most patients had a pretty good idea where their infection came from—and, sadly, whom they might have infected. A caveat here is the fact that it is hard to track the spread of a virus when you cannot locate patient zero because they never presented to a health-care facility with symptoms.

With more data at our fingertips, we could trace back most cases to the source of illness and determine whether it was an asymptomatic carrier, which would in turn help with future prevention. The over-whelming majority (81 percent) of symptomatic patients with the virus have mild illness (cough, sore throat, fever, myalgia).[7] These symptoms are not specific to COVID-19 but can be seen with many other viral illnesses. This is why testing became so crucial. Testing also ran the gamut of availability, from more rare than hen's teeth to a multiplicity of testing types, including drive-through and rapid test kits mailed to every home. We have ample tests now, and most regulators have ceased requiring them for travel, but they were hard to come by in the early days.

Doctors were (and are) reasonably able to presume someone had COVID-19 if they became short of breath about one week after the onset of the above mild symptoms. We could not rely solely on the presence of a fever because it does not happen in every case, and it is not a common presenting symptom. Cough is the most common presenting symptom; about 50 percent of all COVID-19 patients have one.[7] Additional symptoms specific to this illness in-clude loss of smell and/or taste and reddish-purple nodules on the tips of digits. The latter occurs mostly in children and young adults.

Early to mid 2020, severe disease was reported in 14 percent of patients, most of whom were admitted to the hospital with dyspnea (shortness of breath), hypoxia (oxygen deficiency in body tissue), or greater than 50 percent of lung involvement (when most of the lung is infected with illness).[7] Critical cases accounted for 5 percent of patients, meaning either respiratory failure, shock, or multi-organ dysfunction.[7] Severely and critically ill patients required admission to an intensive care unit (ICU) unit with multispecialist care and most commonly developed a secondary infection—pneumonia. Secondary illnesses are those that present after an initial disease, are usually bacterial in nature, and require treatment with antibiot-ics. (As a teaching physician, I cannot resist this teaching moment. Bacterial infections require antibiotics; viral infections need sleep, hydration, over-the-counter comfort medicines, and distance from other people. Perhaps this can become part of general health aware-ness postpandemic.)

So back to the virus, which now is replicating like mad within the infected person, causing that inflammation discussed earlier. Inflammation makes it difficult for our body to function as it normally would. A patient at this level of disease progression would present with many of the common symptoms: fever, sore throat, and cough. Inside the body, white blood cells are attacking any sort of substances that have become trapped in the mucus membranes of the body, viral or otherwise. Mucus is a normal substance our bodies create to help protect us from pathogens. Its inherent properties will be changed as white blood cells fight off pathogens; mucus becomes thicker with dead cells and viruses. This thickened mucus does not allow for the exchange of oxygen in the lungs very well. That decrease in oxygen exchange is part of the reason patients become hypoxic, or short of breath. When there is decreased oxygen exchange, the body will work harder to breathe, which is taxing over long periods. Our bodies compensate to a point, until they are no longer able to sustain the compensation. This is part of why ventilators were so important in fighting COVID.

From here forward, rapid decrease in functionality occurs unless interventionist medicine assistance combines with the person's body to reverse course. Once the body becomes too tired to breathe, respiratory failure happens and we have to place patients on mechanical ventilation. It was taking two or three weeks, sometimes even longer, for patients to come off ventilators in the ICU.[7] In addition to the danger of additional bacterial infections like pneumonia, some patients developed low blood pressure and required medications to increase it. As blood pressure drops, organs start to fail because they are not receiving the required nutrients or blood flow to function. Heart failure and kidney failure are common among patients in the ICU with COVID-19. For those who make it, the road to recovery is slow, exhausting, and may include lasting effects from the disease.

Anyone admitted to an ICU on ventilation or with a serious illness will take weeks, even months to recuperate. For each day an individual is in the ICU, estimate three to five days of physical and occupational therapy to recover back to their baseline functioning.

Some individuals will recover completely with no lasting effects; others become "long haulers," the nickname given COVID-19 patients who "recover" yet show continued systemic illness; long haulers are still under close scrutiny for emergent patterns, but some require lifelong oxygen or even dialysis, among other effects.[7] Identifying all the lasting effects of serious COVID illness will continue for years as we morph from the pandemic to the endemic stage of this coronavirus, because each sequela takes time to present itself.

The one constant of fighting this pandemic has been how rapidly information changes. Some of the information has stabilized and coalesced into protocols for containing this virus and its variants. Like the flu, COVID will be an endemic and unwelcome guest in our lives for years to come. Like the flu, good hygiene and smart medicine can minimize its negative effects in our personal lives and our communities.

Yet comparisons to flu can be misleading, because COVID-19 is a different illness than we are used to, and by "we" in this instance, I mean both medical professionals and the general public. The flu is no longer novel, and we have a vaccine available each year to take to prevent severe illness. Time will tell whether COVID will require annual boosters or if those with three to four vaccinations and boosters under their belt (or should I say, in their arm) will be protected for life.

Back to those comparisons: when someone catches the flu, the onset of symptoms is rapid. You will get a fever, develop chills and muscle aches, and then usually improve within a week. COVID-19 metes out a slower, more nonspecific onset of symptoms. One of the most dangerous and frustrating aspects of this illness was how many patients told us later, sometimes just before ventilation and with tears in their eyes, that in those early stages of feeling mildly ill, they decided they could not have had COVID. This might be because they had stayed home most of the time and had worn their mask while in public, or because they "always get sick this time of year." It was pollen, it was exhaustion, it was never COVID in anyone's mind—until it was. This was even more true after vaccinations began. How could one who had done everything right still get COVID?

Once patients became ill enough to be aware that their self-diagnosed seasonal cold or allergy was actually COVID-19, it was too late to prevent viral spread to others. Patients in serious distress were dealing with guilt at infecting others—naming friends and family they could have infected, and crying—just at a time when they most needed to concentrate all their thoughts, prayers, and positivity on getting well. Of all the effects of the pandemic on health-care providers, watching this pattern repeat was among the most heartbreaking.

### COVID AND THE ELDERLY

Another heartbreaking effect was the loneliness of the elderly caused by the virus and the essential policies put in place to prevent spread. One of the few certainties about COVID as the summer of 2020 morphed into fall was that elderly patients and those with comorbidities (other chronic illnesses) had a much higher risk of severe and critical presentations of the disease and death. Such comorbidities include heart disease, sugar diabetes, high blood pressure, chronic lung disease, cancer, chronic kidney disease, obesity, and smoking. The average number of comorbidities in patients who died from COVID-19 proved to be 2.7 illnesses.[4]

Once a compromised patient was hospitalized with SARS-CoV-2, certain laboratory findings suggested, their doctors and family could expect difficult outcomes. Knowing early on how much more deadly the illness was to these specific populations helped develop prediction tools. Unfortunately, there was a learning curve in attaining evaluation and validation for clinical management.[4] Each case of COVID-19 that came through the doors of an emergency room or ICU was different, and as physicians taking care of these patients, we adjusted accordingly.

In the United States, 80 percent of COVID deaths prior to vaccination occurred in individuals 65 and older.[4] Why is this virus so much more deadly to the elderly? Is it because they are more likely to have comorbidities, or is there some other underlying factor? We know this virus attacks the lungs and can cause coagulopathies (increased risk of developing blood clots). We also know the elderly have decreased lung function and are at increased risk of coagulopathies, pandemic or not. Frailty may also come into play because, as described above, fighting serious cases of any illness takes a huge toll on the body. COVID is certainly no exception. Information slowly emerged about better COVID survival among elderly patients in good health with highly active lifestyles. Lifestyle, psychological, and social factors affect whether someone will contract a viral illness once exposed—any virus, including COVID.[8] When a person has a more active lifestyle, good social structure, and healthy habits, their chance of contracting viral illness decreases. Avoiding worry and guilt during serious infections will also help. All this explains, perhaps, why COVID was such a killer, given the early days of fear, uncertainty, and isolation in the face of this new disease.

A colleague in my emergency room once said in a moment of angry sadness that COVID-19 found all the cracks in our American way of life and inserted its protein spikes into them so it would live forever. That remains true in our current societal attitudes toward hygiene, healthy eating, and exercise; in health outcomes among different races and ethnic communities; and even in family cohesion regarding the elderly. Older people are often isolated by physical conditions that make it tedious or impossible to leave the home. Pandemic restrictions on visitation of the elderly meant they lost a key component of mental wellness to help fight off illness. Perhaps that was the ultimate catch-22 in caring for our elders during the pandemic. Elders are at highest risk of catching and dying from the disease, but using mental positivity and social interaction (both proven health benefits in disease prevention) could result in them getting infected.

How does social isolation contribute to decreased ability to fight off infection? Positive social interaction with people we love has an overall constructive effect on our health regardless of age. Being at home and socially isolated causes loneliness and increases stress. Respect for elders in its truest sense meant protecting them while making sure their other needs were met. As humans we needed to show more compassion, not only during the time of this pandemic, but every day. People learned to check in on parents, grandparents, neighbors, and friends without actually dropping in. Churches set up phone call brigades and organized grocery drop-offs for those who lost work or lived outside an order-online service area. Even though those protein spikes tried to insert themselves into the cracks in our way of life, some amazing ingenuity and kindness emerged as well. This is a good lesson for us all to learn as we continue to incorporate changes into our daily lives, even as we emerge slowly from the pandemic.

### HOW IS SARS-COV-2 DIAGNOSED?

Diagnosis of any disease starts with a history and physical examination. COVID-19 proved no different from any other illness in that regard. Presenting symptoms and patient history helped determine if someone should be tested for the illness, especially when tests were hard to find and cases were rising by the literal minute. Anyone symptomatic should have been tested because there could not be a definitive diagnosis without microbiologic testing. Of course, this was not always possible. Doctors also used presentation and other factors, which is why even now getting correct data on the actual number of people infected, death rates, and recovery rates of the illness remains so debated. And at the hyperlocal level, in order to get the patient in front of us correctly charted, coded for coverage, and treated, we needed completed tests.

Testing was also essential for asymptomatic people prior to surgical procedures, after close prolonged contact with another person infected with COVID-19, among hospitalized patients in an area where community spread was feasible, prior to patients receiving immunosuppressive therapy (such as preparatory to an organ transplant), and among individuals living in long-term care facilities, correctional facilities, and homeless shelters. Testing asymptomatic people in the community, when it could be done, helped determine asymptomatic rates and community spread. This improved as 2020 moved into 2021, but in the early stages, it was something akin to a nightmare.

Also, this sort of testing would usually be conducted by health departments throughout the country.[9] As we know, once enough test kits were available, they were mailed to homes to try and ease the overburdened system. Comprehensive testing of asymptomatic people would also have given us a better picture of case and death rates. Several different types of testing exist; now we are spoiled for choice and the most contentious point of testing is which insurance companies will pay for it.

The polymerase chain reaction (PCR) test is the preferred method because of its sensitivity, correctly detecting when the disease is present 71–98 percent of the time.[10] Some localities will use an antigen test, which is not as sensitive as the PCR test. Obtaining specimens could also be done in multiple ways: a nasopharyngeal swab (similar to an influenza swab), a nasal swab (inner portions of both nostrils are swabbed), nasal or nasopharyngeal aspirates (done in hospital settings), or an oropharyngeal swab (similar to swabbing for strep throat). Initial studies stated that nasal and nasopharyngeal swabs were more sensitive than oral swabs, but data at the time of writing finds that oral/saliva specimens are just as accurate (another example of the minute-by-minute updates doctors received about how to deliver the best possible care against this novel virus).

If an antigen test returned negative, a PCR test could help the patient avoid a false negative. PCR tests were less likely to return false results, but if one came back negative amid high suspicion the patient had the illness, repeat testing would be done when available, after waiting at least 24–48 hours. The sensitivity of the PCR test depends on the type and quality of the specimen obtained, duration of illness at the time of testing, and the specific assay.[9] All that is just a fancy way of saying the swab needs to get enough viral particles, the person being swabbed has to have enough viral particles in their nose at the time of testing, and the lab has to process it correctly in order to have good results.

Along with the PCR and antigen tests, a serologic (blood) antibody test could identify people with prior or late infection. Finding out you had COVID by testing months later might be useful now, or merely interesting. It was not much help during our fight to contain the virus. It is almost impossible to imagine anyone in the United States, or any other country, who does not know someone who had COVID-19. It is inevitable.

## TREATMENT

You're going to read this next part as if we were still in the depths of the pandemic. Think of it like a time capsule, because in order to understand how we felt and what we did as doctors, you need to be in the moment with us. So reset your mind to around September 2020: the virus was raging, the vaccines were nowhere in sight, and we had no idea how long this would last. Ready? Come with me down this nightmare alley of memory lane.

Unlike prevention, where individual choices can make a difference, once a person has COVID the virus begins calling the shots, by which I mean that treatment depended on the severity of the person's illness. If a person is stable and healthy with no comorbidities, they will be advised to stay home and keep their primary care physician apprised of any worsening symptoms. If a person is unstable (extremely short of breath, has low blood pressure, etc.) they will be placed in the hospital, assuming there were available beds. Some hospitals had been overwhelmed with COVID patients while others looked like ghost towns, and then the pendulum would swing and the virus would surge in that ghost town as the overwhelmed hospital eased off. If a hospital was at maximum capacity, patients got transferred to another available hospital. This is called hospital diversion and happens in normal circumstances; because geographic areas tended to be hot spots at the same time, rural areas sometimes made out better than cities in sending patients to other places. That part was unusual. The availability of a bed not only depended on the physical bed being present but having sufficient staff and machinery to take care of the patient. Some locations turned entire hospitals into COVID-specific hospitals, if others were available for general care.

Once in the hospital, patients were either placed in a COVID unit or put into COVID-ICU. From there the treatment varied widely according to the physician taking care of these patients and a patient's presentation of symptoms. Some only required supplemental oxygen, while others needed intravenous antibiotics (because they developed pneumonia or other infections), invasive ventilation, dialysis, and even ECMO (a machine that replaces the function of the heart and lungs). This depended on their level of personal health before infection, the viral load they received at infection, and comorbidities. (Permit me to put in a plug here: viral load is another reason to wear masks; even if you get infected, you will get less of a viral load at the time, which helps you combat the illness if your body succumbs.)

When a patient admitted to the hospital with severe respiratory illness does not have a definite diagnosis of COVID-19, doctors put them on empiric antibiotics (an antibiotic that treats most common bacterial causes of suspected illness) for community acquired pneumonia. The two illnesses are difficult to distinguish from one another until testing has returned. Patients hospitalized with COVID-19 were started on medications to prevent blood clots. Many studies had already shown a high rate of blood clots among hospitalized COVID patients.[11]

Nonsteroidal medications (used to treat pain and inflammation) and nebulized medications (breathing treatments) needed to be avoided because they seemed to make the patient worse. Nebulized medications could cause aerosolization of the virus, which is dangerous to health-care workers. When needed, these were given via inhalers. Hospitalists also tried to avoid medications that suppress the immune system, but they needed to weigh the risks and benefits to each patient. Doctors sometimes opted to give a patient a medication that suppresses the immune system (corticosteroid) to help reduce inflammation in the lungs and other areas. When more and more physicians started using corticosteroids regularly on COVID patients, they noticed patients started to improve. Multiple randomized trials would eventually bear out this observational data, but at the time we were simply flinging emails at each other: "Try this!"

There were many specific treatments under trial, some more infamous than others: steroids (specifically dexamethasone), antivirals (remdesivir), convalescent plasma (plasma from people that had COVID and survived), and hydroxychloroquine, just to name a few. The popularity of monoclonal antibodies rose and fell as data honed their use to specific comorbidities and types of infection. The role of steroids is to reduce the inflammation that comes with the illness. The RECOVERY Trial was a multicenter, randomized, open-label trial in hospitalized patients with severe disease that proved there was benefit to administering steroids (dexamethasone) during treatment.[12] Steroids do have immunosuppressive activity, so this needed to be taken into consideration when administering it to patients.

Remdesivir became something patients learned to ask for by name as COVID information solidified in both hospital best practice and public opinion. Remdesivir was initially designed to treat hepatitis C and RSV, and Gilead, the company that created the antiviral, found it had other possible applications in addition to targeting those two viruses. It works by preventing the viruses from making more copies of themselves. In previous crises, small trials were conducted to see if it could treat SARS, MERS, and Ebola, but sample sizes were too small to generate good data. COVID-19 had a much larger sample size worldwide, and remdesivir is now suggested for hospitalized patients who are not on ventilators or other life support measures.[11]

Convalescent plasma and antibody therapies got significant air time in American media. Providing patients currently sick with plasma from those who had recovered introduced ready-made antibodies for COVID-19, especially for individuals whose bodies cannot mount a good response to the illness on their own. Early research showed that administering this plasma to severely ill patients did reduce the number of RNA particles in the patient's nasopharyngeal swabs, but there was no statistically significant clinical improvement when compared to placebo and standard care.[13] Two full years after the pandemic began, this method continues to be hotly debated.

Hydroxychloroquine became arguably the most political of the trial treatments. Its proposed mechanism of action against the virus was through increasing the pH of endosomes and lysosomes (transportation mechanisms in the cells of our bodies), making it difficult for the virus to replicate because the virus uses that same machinery to produce copies of itself. Hydroxychloroquine has been around for many years, used to treat malaria, lupus, rheumatoid arthritis, and other immunologic illnesses. Studies used this medication to treat SARS-CoV-2, but no statistically significant evidence showed that it decreased mortality or shortened the course of the illness if not used in the first stages of illness. Trials had also been conducted in conjunction with azithromycin (an antibiotic), and the results still had not shown a benefit. Some doctors advocated its use prophylactically for individuals in the medical field and those that have been in contact with someone who was confirmed to have the illness, but evidence of its benefit is inconclusive, or minimally beneficial at best. Also, its use alone or in conjunction with azithromycin did lead to some increase in adverse events, including heart arrhythmias.[14] This is not an unknown or new side effect; hydroxychloroquine has always been cautioned against for individuals with known arrhythmia, among other issues.

Politically, this drug could not catch a break. Media portrayals of hydroxychloroquine as a big bad medication were as incorrect as touting it as a miracle cure for the COVID infected. Hydroxychloroquine is used every day by millions of people worldwide and has side effects just as any other medication does. Politics and medicine are not comfortable hospital bedfellows.

Ivermectin was another medication under hot debate for the treatment of COVID-19. This medication has been used safely for many years to treat tropical diseases such as onchocerciasis, helminthiases, and scabies in humans (just to correct the false idea that it is solely a sheep or horse dewormer). Currently, it is not approved by the Food and Drug Association for the treatment of any viral infection, but it was tested in humans through randomized trials and cohort studies. In vitro studies showed ivermectin did reduce viral replication, but the dose needed to treat humans would be 100-fold the current recommended (safe) dose of this medication. When a safe dose (400 µg/kg) of ivermectin was given, these trials/studies concluded ivermectin had no benefit when used to treat COVID-19 infections. For this reason, the CDC has recommended against its use in the treatment of COVID-19.[15]

INFECTION CONTROL AND PREVENTION

Okay, let's leave our time capsule behind and return to the present day. Most of us are familiar with the old proverb that an ounce of prevention is worth a pound of cure, and nowhere could this have been wiser advice than in the COVID-19 pandemic. Initially, the American people and those worldwide were advised to take shelter in their home for 14 days to slow the spread of the disease and to prevent overwhelming the health-care systems of the world (like what happened almost immediately after this advice was issued in Italy). This was called, back in those naive, optimistic days, "flattening the curve." It did not work; compliance, fear, confusion, mixed messages—many factors contributed to the spiking of the curve in at least four COVID infection rate waves.

Six months after the initial "this will all be over in a couple of weeks" phase, we were still strongly encouraged to stay home; some states lifted and others continued the quarantine mandates. Small businesses closed, while Amazon, Walmart, Target, Lowe's, and Home Depot continued to function with one-way aisles and limits on the number of shoppers—and, hopefully, masks, although this ranged widely.

Decades from now, people will still debate the wisdom of mask and vaccine mandates, why some places were closed and others were allowed to remain open, and how messaging was handled. Unfortunately, those debates were no help in the midst of case counts rising and ebbing, only to rise again with new variants. To stop the spread, the world looked for a vaccine, which began rolling out in November 2020 in the United States.

Meanwhile, as a doctor, I debated yet another dilemma. I work in an area where poverty runs rampant, where $25,000 per year is considered a good salary. While costs of living may be lower in my region, $25K does not offer a lot of savings margins. Hence, keeping businesses closed with no relief package in sight caused additional stresses and hardships on an already-burdened population. Shutting down helped us save lives, but it also threw many people into desperate situations with additional stressors. There was no way to win. Perhaps my emergency department colleague was right; the cracks in our way of life let the virus in to wreak havoc. Long-haul COVID is bad enough; the long-haul devastation to Appalachia's economy because of COVID cannot be overestimated. What health effects will that have on our communities?

Let us not forget mental health, or even physical safety, in that tally. Child and domestic abuse calls went down, but experts in those fields suggested incidences were going up; unemployment went up and down in essential and nonessential working venues. These were the effects of the pandemic outside of the clinics and hospitals. All too soon, we saw them inside. Social determinants of health never left us when the pandemic took over; the cracks are wider now and easier to see, when poverty stresses a family to the breaking point.

### THE MORE THINGS CHANGE

We all remember how governors of each state used a combination of restrictions to help slow the spread of this virus: social distancing orders, stay-at-home orders, school/venue/nonessential business closures, bans on public gatherings, travel restriction, aggressive case identification and isolation, and contact tracing and quarantine.[4] Some proved more successful than others, but no state, town, or community remains unscathed. In addition, the November 2020–January 2021 holiday season saw exponential explosions of caseloads as people just got tired of staying home and not seeing loved ones. That time period became the largest spike of COVID cases and deaths we had seen up to that point. Omicron would later wipe out this dubious achievement, yet even in December 2021, cases of the omicron variant were climbing while deaths remained low; when vaccination and antibody levels go up, deaths go down.

I mentioned before how often the virus was described as hitting in waves, but think of it for a moment like a patchwork quilt; it spread quickly over communities and either spiked rapidly or boiled slowly under the surface, spreading consistently over a longer period of time. Sometimes the quilt warms you quickly; other times you curl up and lie beneath it, slowly getting warmed.

In December 2020, the US was experiencing massive infection rates exceeding 200,000 new cases per day. That number declined by May 2021, with one-third of adult Americans having at least one vaccination dose. At the time of this writing, more than a year later, every American willing to be has been fully vaccinated and boosted. According to data gathered by CNN, an average of seven doses per day continue to be given out worldwide, with population coverage rates ranging from closing in on 100 percent in the United Arab Emirates and Brunei, with Samoa right behind at 99 percent, down to Yemen and Haiti hovering around 1.5 percent.[16]

Vaccines take time to create, study, and put through trials; the Pfizer, Moderna, and Johnson & Johnson vaccines were debated hotly in public opinion yet underwent rigorous testing; they just went through that testing faster, an important distinction. Information readily available online at the CDC includes the current vaccination rates of Americans by age group in an up-to-date format. America is not yet at 100 percent, but odds are good that we have vaccinated everyone willing to be. Check out the numbers for yourself.

⏝

In this pandemic, after so many lives have been lost, everyone is more aware of their health and those around them. Applications to medical school are up. In my position as faculty for an Appalachian residency program, I look forward to seeing more local applications from those inspired by the pandemic to become part of a long-term solution. Perhaps COVID-19's legacy will not be remembered as burning down the house so much as sparking a fire in a future

researcher who will find the cure for the common cold—and in accountability demands for just how long trials should realistically
take to approve a vaccine or drug. Perhaps we have begun a research
journey to find the cure for all cancers. The public has never been
so keenly aware of the need for research, clinical trials, and answers.
Not to mention how often we should wash our hands.

This is what humanity does: rebuild, learn, and change for the
better. If nothing else, this and former pandemics show that we are
built for survival. We are the masters of our fate, no longer victims of
those tiny invaders that can only be seen with a microscope—because
we have the scientific knowledge to see to its undoing and the social compassion to use that knowledge wisely. Perhaps 100 percent
agreement is not achievable. But health is.

### REFERENCES

1 Bramanti, B., Dean, K.R., Walløe, L., Chr Stenseth, N. The Third
   Plague pandemic in Europe. *Proceedings, Biological Sciences*
   2019;286(1901). doi:10.1098/rspb.2018.2429.
2 Cartwright, M. Black Death. Ancient History Encyclopedia,
   March 28, 2020. https://www.ancient.eu/Black_Death/.
3 Jordan, D., Tumpey, T., Jester, B. The deadliest flu: the complete story of the discovery and reconstruction of the 1918 pandemic virus.
   Centers for Disease Control and Prevention, December 17, 2019.
   https://www.cdc.gov/flu/pandemic-resources/reconstruction-1918
   -virus.html.
4 McIntosh, K. COVID-19: epidemiology, virology, and prevention. UpToDate. https://www.uptodate.com/contents/covid-19
   -epidemiology-virology-and-prevention. Accessed May 31, 2022.
5 Institut national de la recherche scientifique (INRS). Common cold
   viruses reveal one of their strengths: the evolution of alphacorona-
   viruses. ScienceDaily, November 27, 2017. www.sciencedaily.com
   /releases/2017/11/171127105937.htm.
6 Goldman, E. Exaggerated risk of transmission of COVID-19 by fo-
   mites. *Lancet;*2020;20:892–893. https://www.thelancet.com/pdfs
   /journals/laninf/PIIS1473-3099(20)30561-2.pdf.
7 COVID-19 can wreck your body, here's how. Nebraska Medicine,
   July 7, 2020. https://www.nebraskamed.com/COVID/what-the
   -coronavirus-does-to-your-body.

8 Cohen, S. Psychosocial vulnerabilities to upper respiratory infectious illness: implications for susceptibility to coronavirus disease 2019 (COVID-19). Perspectives on Psychological Science, July 8, 2020. doi:10.1177/1745691620942516.

9 Caliendo, A.M., and Hanson, K.E. COVID-19: diagnosis. UpToDate. https://www.uptodate.com/contents/covid-19-diagnosis. Accessed May 31, 2022.

10 Watson, J., Whiting, P.F., Brush, J.E. Interpreting a COVID-19 test result. BMJ. 2020;369:m1808. https://www.bmj.com/content/369/bmj.m1808.

11 Kim, A.Y., Gandhi, R.T. Coronavirus disease 2019 (COVID-19): management in hospitalized adults. UpToDate. https://www.uptodate.com/contents/covid-19-management-in-hospitalized-adults. Accessed May 31, 2022.

12 RECOVERY Collaborative Group, Horby, P., Lim, W.S, Emberson, J.R., Mafham, M., et al. Dexamethasone in hospitalized patients with COVID-19—preliminary report. New England Journal of Medicine., 2021;384:693–704. doi:10.1056/nejmoa2021436.

13 Ling, L., Zhang, W., Hu, Y., et al. Effect of convalescent plasma therapy on time to clinical improvement in patients with severe and life-threatening COVID-19. Jama. 2020;324:460. doi:10.1001/jama.2020.10044.

14 Cavalcanti, A.B., Zampieri, F.G., Rosa, R.G., et al. Hydroxychloroquine with or without azithromycin in mild-to-moderate COVID-19. New England Journal of Medicine. 2020;383:2041–2052. doi:10.1056/nejmoa2019014.

15 Ivermectin. COVID-19 treatment guidelines. National Institutes of Health, last updated April 29, 2022. https://www.covid19treatmentguidelines.nih.gov/therapies/antiviral-therapy/ivermectin/.

16 Holder, J. Tracking coronavirus vaccinations around the world. New York Times, updated August 15, 2022. https://www.nytimes.com/interactive/2021/world/covid-vaccinations-tracker.html.

# 3

## The Perfect Storm, the Perfect Solution?

*COVID-19 and Telehealth*

KATHY HSU WIBBERLY

*Editor's Note: Delivering health care through technology has been around for decades, but nothing accelerated its use or cleared policy barriers like the pandemic. Keep in mind the background of the first chapter on rural hospital challenges as you read, and consider the tertiary effects of telehealth take-up on clinics and hospitals in rural areas. Has delivery of medicine changed—for good?*

In the blink of an eye, the pandemic made telehealth and health care synonymous. Nobody wanted to go near an actual clinic or doctor, let alone an actual hospital. At the same time, doctors recognized the seismic shift that had just occurred in how medicine would be delivered over the next year, if not decade. While it may seem as if telehealth has become an overnight sensation, the reality is that this mode of service delivery has a 30-year history.

The terms *telemedicine* and *telehealth* are sometimes seen as synonymous. *Telehealth* refers broadly to the use of electronic information and telecommunications technologies to support remote clinical health care, patient and professional health-related education, public health, and health administration. *Telemedicine* is a subset of telehealth and specifically refers to the use of such technologies for direct clinical care between a patient and a health-care provider.

In *Understanding Telehealth* (2018), Thomas S. Nesbitt and Jana Katz-Bell, both from the UC Davis School of Medicine, coauthored a chapter on the "History of Telehealth" that stated "the 1990s came to be regarded as the 'developmental years' of telemedicine" and that this was the decade during which many large state and health system telehealth initiatives began to emerge. There were two primary drivers for this. First, broadband telecommunications became more readily available and affordable. Dial-up connection came into being during the 1980s, and at that time it was considered cutting-edge technology. Those who were part of the dial-up generation will recall with some sense of nostalgia the sound of the modem dialing the phone number to an internet service provider and the screeching sound that happened when the connection was made. They might also wag their fingers at the younger generation, sharing tales (with perhaps a sense of pride and accomplishment) of how incredibly slow the connection was, allowing a person time to go make a cup of coffee or a sandwich while waiting for a single web page to load.

During the 1990s, we rejoiced to see the gradual transition from dial-up to high-speed internet—what we now call broadband—across most of the United States. (Some rural areas do not yet have broadband access.) While still slow by today's standards, broadband at least made a reasonable video connection plausible. Soon after, passage of state and federal legislation propelled the field forward by recognizing telemedicine as a reimbursable mode of care provision—a real game changer.

Nesbitt and Bell discussed how the field of telemedicine matured from 2000 to 2009 with the growth of what has traditionally been called a "hub-and-spoke" network model (see fig. 3.1). In this model, a larger tertiary care facility (one that a primary care doctor refers a patient to for care from specialists) typically contracts with smaller community-based clinics and hospitals to provide specialty care services using telehealth technologies. The nice thing about this model is that patients get to stay in their home community while getting care from specialists. As an additional perk, this model facilitated better communication between primary care providers and

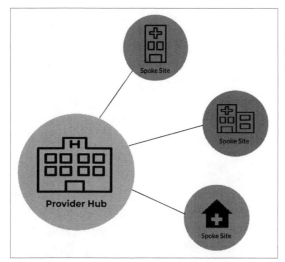

FIG. 3.1. Hub-and-spoke network model.

specialists. Examples of well-established hub-and-spoke models of telemedicine that started up in the 2000s include telestroke, telepsychiatry, teledermatology, and telecardiology.

The next decade (beginning in 2010 and ending just before the start of the COVID-19 pandemic) arrived with the implementation of the Affordable Care Act (ACA). In 2008, the Centers for Medicare & Medicaid Services (CMS) began emphasizing value-based care (that is, care that rewards health-care providers with incentive payments based on the quality of care they provide) over volume-based or fee-for-service care (where payments are associated with the quantity of encounters and procedures). The ACA authorized a number of value-based care incentive programs when it was implemented in 2010. Additionally, by 2010, over 65 percent of US households had broadband services.

As CMS started steering the direction of health care from volume-based to value-based care, wireless network technology (Wi-Fi) was becoming the standard for connecting to the internet. The idea of connected ("smart") devices has been around for a long time; the term *Internet of Things* (IoT) was coined by Kevin Ashton in 1999 during his work at Procter & Gamble. The actual concept in implementation did not start gaining popularity until 2010. Instead of humans communicating with each other, IoT envisioned a system of internet-connected gadgets being able to collect and transfer data over a wireless network without the need for human intervention. In health care, this opened up the entire universe of wearable devices, sensors, and more.

The convergence of national health-care reform with significant advancements in speed and multitasking ability for both broadband infrastructure and telehealth technologies created an environment that was ripe for expansion of telemedicine beyond the hub-and-spoke model to a distributed network model. In a distributed network, any facility and any individual can connect with any other health-care facility or provider.

Distributed networks opened up the world of health care to applications that went beyond telemedicine to those under the broader umbrella of telehealth. Popular examples of this broader definition include initiatives like Project ECHO, eConsults, and Remote Patient Monitoring.

Project ECHO (Extension for Community Healthcare Outcomes) was launched in 2003 as an outgrowth of the frustration experienced by Sanjeev Arora, MD, a liver disease specialist at the University of New Mexico Health Sciences Center in Albuquerque. Arora found he had the capacity to serve only a fraction of the hepatitis C patients in the state who needed his services. In an effort to expand his reach, he developed a telementoring model and offered it free of charge for community providers across New Mexico. The telementoring model leverages telehealth technologies to support interactive dialogue, comanagement of cases, peer-to-peer learning and collaborative problem solving. By enhancing the knowledge, skills, and confidence of community providers, patients of family providers or hospitalists can benefit from care mentored by specialists at a university. This program model has rapidly expanded throughout the country and world for an ever-growing number of specialty and subspecialty content areas.

Project ECHO is a synchronous provider-to-provider and peer-to-peer telementoring model that connects community providers with specialists; eConsults serves a similar function in an asynchronous manner. (Applications of telehealth can take place either synchronously, in real time virtual interactions between parties, or asynchronously, as electronic transmission of digital images, prerecorded videos, and other sources of information and data to be reviewed at a later, more convenient time by one or more parties.) Asynchronous applications of telehealth are also referred to as "store and forward." A common example of an asynchronous telehealth is the transmission of medical images such as X-rays for review by a radiologist. With the eConsult model, community providers use a platform to present patient case information and data for review by a specialist. Specialists review the information when they are available, and if the information is adequate, they return a diagnosis with recommendations for treatment to the community provider. A report summarizing studies of this program model has shown improved access to specialty care, more efficient use of health-care resources, high patient and clinician satisfaction, and lower total cost of care.[1]

Remote patient monitoring (RPM) uses digital technologies to collect medical and other forms of health data from individuals in one location and then transmits that information electronically to health-care providers elsewhere for assessment. These digital technologies range from Bluetooth-enabled peripheral devices to wearable devices to sensors embedded in homes, cars, and even people. By leveraging the IoT concept for health-care purposes, RPM became one of the driving forces behind the shift from episodic care to continuous, proactive whole-person care across the entire care continuum. The ability to monitor patients no matter their location moved the needle on the concepts of "care anywhere," "health care without walls," and "direct-to-consumer," or DTC, telehealth services. DTC services refer to health-care services provided to the patient at the patient's request either immediately on demand or at a scheduled time in the future, without the patient having to travel to a particular location for that care.

## SLOW AND STEADY GROWTH

While telehealth's use has seen relatively steady growth over the past 30 years, that growth prepandemic was mostly linear. Telehealth within hospital and emergent care settings has had the most time to come to maturity; its use has advanced more rapidly (from roughly 54 percent in 2014 to approximately 71 percent in 2017, according to the Healthcare Information and Management Systems Society [HIMSS] Analytics 2017 Inpatient Telemedicine Essentials Brief Snapshot Report). Adoption of telehealth in the outpatient setting lags well behind. This is particularly true in private practice.

Deloitte is a privately held company that tracks and monitors trends through survey research. In 2018, Deloitte conducted a survey of US physicians and found the following:

> Nine in 10 physicians see the benefits of virtual care. . . .
> Current levels of implementation are low. Forty-four
> percent of surveyed physicians have not implemented
> any of the seven virtual care technologies presented
> in the survey. The technology implemented most so
> far is email/patient portal consultations (38 percent),
> followed by physician-to-physician electronic consulta-
> tions (17 percent), and virtual/video visits (14 percent).
> For the remaining four of the seven technologies in the
> survey—remote care management and coaching, remote
> patient monitoring at home, remote patient monitoring
> at other facilities, and integration of wearables—reported
> adoption is in single digits.[2]

Slowing growth in the adoption of telehealth by providers is resistance to change—that is, maintaining the status quo and the inability for policy making to keep pace with advances in technology.

The term *status quo bias* was first introduced in 1988 by two researchers at Harvard: William Samuelson and Richard Zeckhauser. In a series of controlled experiments, they found that people showed a disproportionate preference for choices that maintained the status quo. Much could be said in a positive vein about maintaining the status quo, as it is both comfortable and familiar. Why rock the boat when things are going just fine? The status quo for health-care delivery in the United States, until recently, revolved around in-person care. Health-care professionals were trained using this model, and little was done to move beyond.

Another contributor to maintaining the status quo is the slow diffusion of innovation. To better understand issues surrounding the diffusion and adoption of technology, one need only examine the history of the stethoscope, taken from a blog post by the Melnick Medical Museum:

> The practice of percussion and immediate auscultation were popular in physical examinations by the early 1800s. . . . A French physician named Rene Laennec (1781–1826) was a firm believer in this method of diagnosis. He worked to refine the auscultation procedure and link the sounds with specific physiological changes in the chest. Immediate auscultation could be an awkward procedure, particularly for female patients. In 1816, Laennec found himself in one of these situations. He rolled a few sheets of thick paper into a tube shape and applied the tube to the woman's chest instead of his ear. Later, he made a more durable instrument out of wood and called it the stethoscope. It was a monaural model that consisted of one tube and was used on one ear. The first practical bi-aural stethoscope was made in 1851. . . . While many physicians readily adopted monaural stethoscopes, the bi-aural stethoscopes were met with some skepticism. Doctors worried about hearing imbalances caused by using both ears instead of one. For this reason, many doctors continued to use monaural stethoscopes into the early 1900s.[3]

It is hard for modern minds to fathom why it took over 50 years for the stethoscope to become commonplace as a tool in a clinician's practice. The diffusion of innovation (DOI) theory may be useful for shedding light on this enigma. DOI was first proposed in 1962 by Dr. Everett M. Rogers, distinguished professor in the Department of Communication and Journalism at the University of New Mexico. For Rogers, an innovation is an idea, practice, or project that is perceived as new no matter how long that idea, practice, or project has actually been in existence. DOI explains how innovations gain momentum and begin spreading (i.e., diffusing) through a population or social system. The model posits that there are five categories of adopters: innovators, early adopters, early majority, late majority, and laggards.

The diffusion of innovation does not happen simultaneously but starts with the innovators and requires a period of time to move to the other four adopter categories. The majority of the general population falls in the middle categories, so when promoting innovation, different strategies need to be used to appeal to different adopter types.

The DOI is one of the oldest social science theories whose applicability continues to this day. The relevance of DOI is underscored by the 17-year research-to-practice gap borne out of the 2001 Institute of Medicine (now known as the National Academy of Medicine) report entitled "Crossing the Quality Chasm: A New Health System for the 21st Century." The report identified and recommended improvements in six dimensions of health care in the United States: patient safety, care effectiveness, patient centeredness, timeliness, care efficiency, and equity. One finding from the report was that "it now takes an average of 17 years for new knowledge generated by randomized controlled trials to be incorporated into practice." Since that time, efforts have been underway to expedite the process from research into clinical practice, with translational science emerging as a new field of research with this goal in mind. In a 2013 study of contributing factors to the research-to-practice gap within the hospital setting, the researchers concluded that awareness of evidence-based practices alone does not translate into implementation of those practices in the clinical setting.[4] Clinical championship plays a significant role in translating awareness into implementation. In order to become an impetus for culture change over time, the clinical champion needs to be a respected leader who (1) believes that the innovation in practice will benefit both the organization and the patient, (2) exudes enthusiasm, and (3) serves as a role model.

The role of the clinical champion has long been touted as one of the key drivers of success in telehealth program development, and it aligns nicely with modern theories of leading change and change management. Some key tenets for accelerating or leading change include the ability to create a sense of both urgency and opportunity, providing a vision, and being able to convincingly communicate a vision and strategy. While clinical champions can and do emerge at the smaller clinic/private practice environment, it is more difficult than in academic health centers or larger hospital/health system contexts. The latter emphasize both clinical care and research and development. Larger settings also offer tertiary opportunities to be exposed to and challenged by the thoughts and ideas of a greater array of both colleagues and trainees.

The inability of policy making to keep pace with advances in technology is the second contributor to the slow diffusion of telehealth innovation throughout health care. Another key tenet to successfully leading transformation is the ability to remove obstacles from the new vision. The Learning Accelerator (TLA) is a national nonprofit focused on driving innovation in education. 2Revolutions (2Rev) is an organization committed to assisting communities to transform their learning models and systems. In October 2014, Todd Kern (founder and partner, 2Rev) and Lisa Duty (partner, TLA) joined together to research and write a report entitled "So You Think You Want to Innovate? Emerging Lessons and a New Tool for State and District Leaders Working to Build a Culture of Innovation." In this report, they named the policy environment as one of the essential components for establishing a culture of innovation.

Kern and Duty stated that policy environments could be preventive (constraining innovation), permissive (allowing without support), or enabling (actively promoting support and rewarding risk taking). The authors encouraged leaders to actively create more policies aimed at promoting and rewarding innovative behaviors, while stopping those that inhibit innovation.

In the field of telehealth, the culture of innovation has not historically been supported by the policy environment. Over the past several decades, applications of telehealth have multiplied and the technologies being used have experienced rapid growth in their sophistication. However, changes in telehealth policies have been slow to evolve and have not kept up with applications of telehealth or the technologies being used.

The Center for Connected Health Policy identified four barriers to telehealth implementation (see fig. 3.2). Of the four major "buckets" of barriers, three are related to federal and/or state policy and include challenges for reimbursement, licensure, and governing the use of technology. To further complicate the policy landscape, there has been a wide variation across states and little alignment between state and federal policies related to telehealth.

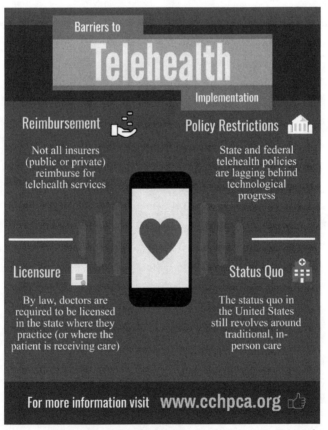

FIG. 3.2. Barriers to telehealth implementation. *Source:* Center for Connected Health Policy, Mei Kwong.

FROM LINEAR TO EXPONENTIAL GROWTH

Ultimately, disruption of the status quo happens in two ways. Either a leader, such as a clinical champion, can choose to disrupt it in order to inspire growth, or life events can disrupt it by making the status quo no longer tenable. The COVID-19 global pandemic was such a disruptor. The COVID-19 pandemic affected patients and health-care providers alike in early March 2020. As news of the coming shutdowns and concerns for viral contagion spread, patients started to cancel in-person appointments at health-care facilities for fear of exposure. At the same time, the anxiety level of health-care providers also increased due to the substantive shortage of personal protective equipment (PPE). To decrease the risk of transmitting the novel coronavirus to patients or health-care workers and to preserve PPE for frontline workers treating those afflicted with COVID-19, health-care practices—sometimes voluntarily and other times by order of state officials—began to defer elective visits. (This is detailed in the following chapter, "Bracing Early for a Delayed Impact.")

The Commonwealth Fund (a private foundation that conducts independent research and supports grant making with the goal of developing high-performing health-care systems for society's most vulnerable populations) closely monitored the impact of COVID-19. They issued a report that looked at the impact of the pandemic on outpatient visits from the start of the pandemic through August 1, 2020: "The number of visits to ambulatory practices fell nearly 60 percent by early April before rebounding through mid-June. From then through the end of July, weekly visits plateaued at 10 percent below the pre-pandemic baseline. The cumulative number of lost visits since mid-March remains substantial and continues to grow."

The perfect storm had arrived, and the world of telehealth was about to expand exponentially. Telehealth was suddenly seen not as a challenge to the status quo or a bane to independent physicians' sovereignty, but as the only viable solution to the challenges brought on by the pandemic.

Funded by the US Department of Health and Human Services Health Resources and the Services Administration Office for the

Advancement of Telehealth for nearly 15 years, Telehealth Resource Centers (TRCs) provide unbiased, nonpartisan, and expert telehealth technical assistance to health-care organizations, networks, and providers. TRCs give advice on how to implement cost-effective telehealth programs, with a particular emphasis on assisting those who work with rural and medically underserved areas and populations. The collective footprint of the 12 regional and 2 national TRCs (see fig. 3.3) reaches across the United States and the affiliated Pacific Islands.

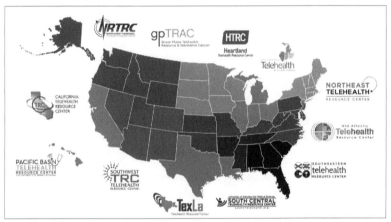

FIG. 3.3. National and Regional Telehealth Resource Centers.

The volume of requests for technical assistance that TRCs receive has historically mirrored the slow but steady linear growth in the adoption of telehealth. To put this in perspective, the number of technical assistance requests in 2019 was 67 percent higher than in 2018 at the Mid-Atlantic Telehealth Resource Center (MATRC). In March 2020, MATRC experienced an 800 percent increase in technical assistance requests (see fig. 3.4).

On a personal note, I wrote these reflections shortly after this peak:

> Now that I've had a decent night's sleep and a few minutes
> to breathe without the phone ringing and the emails ping-
> ing, I just wanted to share a few thoughts from my insane
> week. First, it is amazing that after 30 years, telehealth has

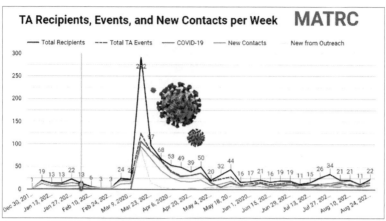

FIG. 3.4. MATRC technical assistance requests per week (December 2019–August 2020).

suddenly become an "overnight" sensation. Please thank one of the many pioneers and champions of telehealth who have tirelessly pressed on developing best practices, training programs, conducting research, pushing the policy and reimbursement envelope, and being willing to innovate with technology to improve care. I can't imagine what would be happening now without all these folks laying the groundwork.

Second, our broadband and cellular infrastructure still sucks. For those of you who don't see internet as a utility and didn't bat an eyelash over the issue of net neutrality, please think again. I spent close to an hour on the phone yesterday with a doctor in a very rural health system. The majority of the patients there do not have internet access in their homes. Some due to cost, others due to lack of available broadband providers and infrastructure. He was really distressed that the telephone was his only means of assessing his patient's conditions . . . not only bad for patient care but not exactly a way to keep a practice running either. In general, physicians are not reimbursed for the time they spend on the phone with patients. In this time of emergency, there have been some provisions made by Medicare and some Medicaid programs, but that rate is around $15. Not exactly a way to keep the lights on in a doctor's office, but better than nothing. A video consult would at least be reimbursed at the office visit rate.

We did a lot of brainstorming. Perhaps he can work with the schools and libraries who do have internet and are currently closed so patients can go there for telehealth consults. Perhaps he can set up a system so patients can stay in their cars and receive a text when the room is available to maintain social distancing and decrease exposure. Perhaps a volunteer could be on-site to wipe down and disinfect the area after each visit. He was actually excited about that possibility. Said he had been working all week on trying to figure out a solution and never thought about using a school or library. I was glad that this gave him some hope, but also really sad that this is where we are in the year 2020.

Third, it isn't just restaurants and small businesses who are at risk of closing their doors. Small private practices are as well since patients are canceling appointments to avoid exposure. There is panic and fear regarding the economic impact in the health-care community that is palpable. One person who was calling, emailing and texting me was bearing the burden of figuring things out for 10 clinicians in very small rural practices. He literally said "About three separate doctors' offices are depending on making telehealth and these telehealth billing codes work to survive this outbreak/pandemic."

Finally, even as many of us have the luxury of working from home and hanging out with families, there are so many in public health who work in hospitals and health systems who are putting in long hours to address COVID-19 and to prepare for the worst. Many are even more stressed by the scarcity of supplies and test kits and having to worry about the constant risk of exposure to

themselves and their families. I think about my daughter
who should be home finishing up her junior year semester
with classes online . . . but instead, because she works as a
scribe in the ED where they have seen multiple COVID-19
cases, is living with a coworker to avoid the risk of exposure to the rest of the family. Who knows how long it will
be before she comes home. There are so many others like
her. They need a kind word, a virtual hug and a thank you
for their sacrifice.

While these stories are in some ways deeply personal and re-
flective of my experience that incredible month, they are also not
unique. Each TRC across the country saw exponential increases in
demand for technical assistance and heard similar stories of fear,
anxiety, compassion, and courage. McKinsey & Company, a global
management consulting firm that works with both private and public health-care leaders, wrote a May 29, 2020, article entitled "Telehealth: A Quarter-Trillion-Dollar Post-COVID-19 Reality?" In that
article, they stated that "COVID-19 has caused a massive acceleration
in the use of telehealth. Consumer adoption has skyrocketed, from
11 percent of US consumers using telehealth in 2019 to 46 percent of
consumers now using telehealth to replace canceled healthcare visits.
Providers have rapidly scaled offerings and are seeing 50 to 175 times
the number of patients via telehealth than they did before."

At the same time that COVID-19 disrupted the status quo,
health-care provider pandemic needs began to shape telehealth policies. It was a tumultuous time on the policy front lines, changes
coming hard and fast. In the first two months, keeping up was nearly
impossible. Providing technical assistance proved particularly challenging, as the correct answer to any particular policy question
could literally be different from one hour to the next. The National
Governors Association wrote the following in its November 2020
report on "The Future of State Telehealth Policy":

It was not until the COVID-19 pandemic reached the
United States that federal, state and commercial payers
created broad flexibility in many telehealth policies to

facilitate physical distancing while maintaining access to
health care services. In addition to providing a mechanism
for individuals to receive care at home, payment parity for
telehealth helped many providers stay solvent during the
COVID-19 pandemic. As a result, there have been more
telehealth policy changes (many of which are temporary)
within the past year than in the past 20 years.

As a reminder, the three federal and/or state policy-related barriers
included challenges around reimbursement, licensure, and policies
that govern the use of technology.

Medicare is the nation's largest payer for health-care services,
but its coverage and reimbursement policies for telehealth had
been extraordinarily restrictive prepandemic. At the end of the
first week of March, Congress passed the Coronavirus Supplemental Appropriations Act (H.R. 6074). This included a $500 million
authorization to enhance telehealth services and also provided the
US Department of Health and Human Services (HHS) with the authority to waive or modify certain telehealth Medicare requirements
during a national or public health emergency (PHE). Prior to the
COVID-19 pandemic and declaration of a PHE, strict restrictions
applied to the traditional Fee-for-Service Medicare program:

- The originating site (location of the patient). Health-care providers could get reimbursed for telehealth services only if
  the Medicare beneficiary was physically located at a specific
  type of facility (e.g., Federally Qualified Health Centers
  [FQHCs], Rural Health Clinics [RHCs], or physician and
  practitioner offices). That facility also had to be located in
  a rural area (county outside of a standard metropolitan
  statistical area) or in a medically underserved census tract
  in a low-population-density area. These restrictions were
  put into place when Medicare Telehealth Services were first
  authorized in the 1990s to address Congressional Budget
  Office concerns and fears about the cost burden that telehealth would place on the Medicare Program. In recent

years, legislators have enabled a handful of exceptions to
these originating site requirements. These exceptions include
treatment for substance use disorder, telestroke, and dialysis
for end-stage renal disease.

- The distant site practitioner (type of provider providing the
telehealth service). Only specific subsets of provider types
were eligible to serve as distant site providers. This included
physicians, nurse practitioners, physician assistants, nurse
midwives, clinical nurse specialists, certified registered nurse
anesthetists, clinical psychologists, clinical social workers,
and registered dietitians or nutrition professionals. FQHCs
and RHCs were specifically excluded from being able to
serve as distant site practitioners. These restrictions were put
into place when Medicare Telehealth Services were first authorized in the 1990s and were a reflection of the types of use
cases that were prevalent at that time. While the landscape of
telehealth use cases has evolved and multiplied, the policies
governing them have not.

- Types of service/procedures. Coverage for telehealth services is
limited to a subset of Current Procedural Terminology (CPT)
or Healthcare Common Procedure Coding System (HCPCS)
procedure codes. In addition, telehealth coverage is only
available for synchronous video-based services. CMS has a
process for providers to submit requests for additional codes
to be considered for coverage each year. In order to meet the
review criteria for consideration, the provider must include
evidence (published and peer reviewed) that the use of telehealth technologies to deliver the proposed service(s) would
be of clinical benefit to the patient. These requirements bump
up against the metaphoric "chicken-and-egg" problem. Telehealth use cases that do not have an adequate reimbursement
mechanism are typically provided by clinicians as small-scale
pilots, sometimes funded through grants. Peer-reviewed
scientific publications, on the other hand, typically require

clinical trials that include diverse populations with large sample sizes. Therefore, it has been exceedingly difficult to meet the review criteria requirements for significantly expanding the list of eligible CPT/HCPCS codes.

On March 17, 2020, CMS released its first set of policy modifications related to telehealth. These were essentially a declaration of regulatory waivers in response to the PHE that then provided the administration the ability to adjust or become more flexible with its telehealth rules and requirements. Many more notices of "flexibilities and waivers" pertaining to telehealth followed over the next days, weeks, and months. The most significant changes to Medicare telehealth services included the following:

- Removal of all of the originating site facility and geographic restrictions. By doing this, it paved the way for patients to be able to receive telehealth services from health-care providers no matter their location, including while at home.

- Removal of distant site practitioner restrictions. While these restrictions were lifted slowly and over time, within about two months of the start of the pandemic all providers who were eligible to bill Medicare for in-person services were also eligible to bill Medicare for those services as distant site providers of telehealth, including physical therapists, occupational therapists, speech language pathologists, FQHCs, and RHCs.

- Expansion of the types of services and procedures allowed to be delivered by telehealth. This list has grown significantly over time and continues to be updated with some regularity. The full list of telehealth eligible CPT/HCPCS codes has more than tripled since the start of the PHE.

- Waiver of the video requirement for evaluation and management (E/M) services and behavioral health counseling and education services. Prior to this waiver, telephone E/M services were not considered telehealth and were thus reimbursed at a lower nontelehealth rate, while behavioral health counseling and education without a video component were not reimbursable services at all. This waiver of the video requirement was put in place in response to the large number of patients who did not have access to broadband, access to devices with video capability, or adequate technology literacy to conduct a video-based telehealth visit. While most providers will acknowledge that video-based care results in better quality of care, there is also a need to balance this with the very real concern about creating disparities in access if providers are not adequately and equitably reimbursed for the time spent on the telephone for patients who do not have other options.

Not long before the pandemic, CMS created a new category of technology-enabled services categorized as Other Virtual Care / Communication Services. Although facilitated through the use of telecommunications technologies, CMS intentionally differentiated these services from their definition of Telehealth (synchronous video-based) Services so that they were not bound by the originating site restrictions associated with Telehealth Services. These Virtual Care / Communication Service billing codes were developed within the context of an established relationship between a primary care provider and a patient.

An example of a Virtual Communication Service is something that CMS calls the "Virtual Check-In." Medicare patients at home may initiate brief communications with their established provider from wherever they are located, including their homes, by telephone, video, secure text messaging, or the use of a patient portal. CMS will reimburse providers for these Virtual Check-Ins so long as the reason is not related to a medical visit within the previous seven days and does not lead to a medical visit within the next 24 hours (or soonest available appointment). Virtual Check-Ins give providers a mechanism to be able to respond to patient concerns, thereby avoiding an unnecessary trip to the provider's office. That became something of a big deal during the pandemic.

As a result of the waivers and flexibilities associated with the PHE, CMS has expanded the types of clinicians who could bill for these

Virtual Care / Communication Services, and they are allowing providers to use these billing codes for both established and new patients.

While CMS regulates coverage and payment policies for Medicare, states have been given significant authority to set their own Medicaid telehealth policy. Typically, states decide what types of restrictions they want to put into place related to telehealth coverage and reimbursement and include those policies in the state plans submitted to CMS for review and approval. As a result, while all state Medicaid programs have been less restrictive than Medicare, if you've seen one state's Medicaid policy, you've seen only one state's Medicaid policy.

In response to the PHE, CMS not only provided waivers and flexibilities pertaining to Medicare but also gave state Medicaid programs broad flexibility to expand coverage for telehealth without having to get federal approval for changes to their state plan. Additionally, CMS allowed states to waive in-person prerequisites associated with a subset of services prior to being able to bill for telehealth services. As with Medicare, state Medicaid programs either eliminated restrictions or significantly expanded their list of eligible originating sites; eligible telehealth distant site providers; list of eligible telehealth services; and list of eligible telehealth modalities (e.g., telephonic visits, synchronous live video visits, remote monitoring, asynchronous store, and forward services).

States also varied significantly in relationship to private insurer coverage for telehealth services. Many but not all states have telehealth parity laws. Such laws restrict private insurers from denying claims solely because services are provided by telehealth. However, most of these parity laws apply only to commercial market plans, not to the self-insured. The lack of uniformity between payers and the wide variation between states contribute to the complexity of navigating telehealth reimbursement policies. This maze of state-by-state scrutiny is one of the reasons why reimbursement policies are cited as a barrier to telehealth.

With the pivot to telehealth by both Medicare and state Medicaid programs, Tricare (the health-care program for uniformed service members, retirees, and their families) and commercial payers also responded to the pandemic with policy adjustments that better supported the use of telehealth services.

In general, a clinician must be licensed in the state where the patient/client is physically located at the time of service. For example, if a provider is licensed in Virginia and sees patients at their office in Northern Virginia, there are no restrictions on patients who live in the District of Columbia or in Maryland coming to the provider's office in Virginia for services. However, if that same patient wanted to remain at home in Maryland and receive telehealth services from the Virginia licensed provider, technically that provider would not be able to see that patient without a Maryland license. Obtaining licenses from multiple states can be tedious and costly, involving paperwork, documentation, meeting of different continuing education requirements, and fees. As a result, many providers saw licensure as a barrier to providing telehealth services.

State licensing boards maintain primary authority for policies related to the licensure of health-care professionals. As a result of the pandemic, many state medical and other health professions' licensing boards created mechanisms that temporarily permitted providers to practice across state lines or expedited processes for licensure and/or recognition of out-of-state licenses. Many states also created mechanisms for providers who are retired and/or have expired licenses to be able to temporarily return to practice.

The Health Insurance Portability and Accountability Act of 1996 (HIPAA) is a federal law that required the creation of national standards to protect sensitive patient health information from being disclosed without the patient's consent or knowledge. HHS issued the HIPAA Privacy Rule to implement the requirements of HIPAA. The Office of Civil Rights within HHS is the regulatory body responsible for ensuring compliance with HIPAA.

On March 30, 2020, the Office of Civil Rights announced that it would exercise enforcement discretion related to HIPAA. This opened the door for individuals and providers to use any available devices with audio and video capabilities (e.g., smartphones and tablets) and any available apps (e.g., Skype and FaceTime) for telehealth visits. Some states also had their own legal requirements pertaining to HIPAA and followed suit by waiving requirements as well.

Needless to say, with the disruption of the status quo and the lifting of policy restrictions, the adoption of telehealth skyrocketed. According to an issue brief looking at the use of telehealth for delivery of primary care services in Fee-for-Service (FFS) Medicare dated July 28, 2020, from the Office of the Assistant Secretary for Planning and Evaluation (ASPE):

- Nearly half of all Medicare primary care visits were via telehealth in April, compared with less than 1 percent in February before the start of the COVID-19 pandemic.

- Based on early experience with Medicare primary care telehealth at the start of the COVID-19 public health emergency, Medicare's new telehealth flexibilities played a critical role in helping to maintain access to primary health-care services.

- The stable and sustained use of telehealth after in-person primary care visits started to resume in mid-April suggests there may be continued demand for telehealth in Medicare, even after the pandemic ends.

According to the Commonwealth Fund (2020) report looking at the impact of the pandemic on outpatient visits, "initially, as in-person visits dropped, telemedicine visits rose rapidly. Since that peak in mid-April, telemedicine use declined, yet appears to have plateaued at a substantially higher rate than prior to the pandemic."

A national poll on healthy aging report looked at telehealth use among older adults before and during COVID-19 and found the following: "In May 2019, 14 percent of older adults said that their health care providers offered telehealth visits, compared to 62 percent in June 2020, while the percentage of older adults who had ever participated in a telehealth visit rose sharply from four percent in May 2019 to 30 percent in June 2020. Of those surveyed in 2020, six percent reported having a telehealth visit prior to March 2020, while 26 percent reported one in the period from March to June 2020."[5]

Finally, according to the McKinsey & Company article, "health systems, independent practices, behavioral health providers and others rapidly scaled telehealth offerings to fill the gap between need and canceled in-person care, and are reporting 50–175 times the number of telehealth visits as pre-COVID. In addition, 57 percent of providers view telehealth more favorably than they did before COVID-19 and 64 percent are more comfortable using it."

### WHERE DO WE GO FROM HERE?

Now that the proverbial genie is out of the bottle, what does the future hold for telehealth? Hundreds of thousands of providers and patients have experienced telehealth for the first time as a result of the pandemic. Early indications show that many health-care providers—not to mention patients—now recognize the value of telehealth and will likely want to continue. The COVID-19 Healthcare Coalition Telehealth Impact Study Work Group analysis of a physician survey administered from July to August 2020 found that more than 75 percent of responding clinicians indicated that telehealth enabled them to provide quality care in the areas of COVID-19-related care, acute care, chronic disease management, hospital follow-up, care coordination, preventative care, and mental/behavioral health. Additionally, 60 percent reported that telehealth had improved the health of their patients.

Sixty-eight percent of respondents are motivated (agree and strongly agree) to increase telehealth use in their practices. The majority would like to continue to offer telehealth for chronic disease management, medical management, care coordination, and preventative care following the pandemic. More than 80 percent of respondents indicated that telehealth improved the timeliness of care for their patients. A similar percentage said that their patients had reacted favorably to using telehealth for care.

Again, according to the McKinsey & Company article, "while the surge in telehealth has been driven by the immediate goal to avoid exposure to COVID-19, with more than 70 percent of in-person visits canceled, 76 percent of survey respondents indicated that they were highly or moderately likely to use telehealth going forward. Also, 74 percent of telehealth users reported high satisfaction."

Providers who made the rapid pivot to telehealth at the start of the pandemic were probably thinking of it as a temporary stopgap measure, but many are starting to count on it as they plan for the future. Fueled in part by the emerging reality of postpandemic life, many health-care systems and individuals are moving toward hybrid care delivery models. While the demand for individual technical assistance requests has decreased since the early weeks of the pandemic, it remains high, averaging a 200–300 percent increase. TRCs have also seen a significant increase in demand for trainings on best practices and requests for tools related to quality measures and sustainability planning. These show that providers are beginning to think longer term, taking steps to fix what I would call "sloppy telehealth."

Sloppy telehealth results from "flying by the seat of your pants" implementation. It is reactive and not proactive. As such, it is not optimal in terms of either efficiency or effectiveness.

Improving telehealth efficiency will require providers to take a step back and to think about why they are using telehealth and what problem(s) they are trying to solve. It will also require practices to identify a clinical champion (or two or three). While many providers have had a positive experience with telehealth as a result of their pandemic-fueled experiences, there will be those who have not. Having a clinical champion will ensure forward momentum and help to institutionalize culture change leading to sustainability. Finally, it will also require providers to think systematically about their program model and workflow. Workflows help to both define and clarify roles and responsibilities. Workflow planning cannot be done in silos but must involve every member of the office or practice. One of the greatest challenges that providers faced when making the rapid pivot to telehealth was transitioning from an in-office workflow where there were defined roles and responsibilities to a telehealth encounter with a patient where both the provider and the patient are disconnected from the rest of the office.

Improving telehealth effectiveness will require a plan for training and retraining. Many providers were truly thrown into the fray and forced to figure their clinical needs out on the fly. Providers can improve their clinical assessment skills, become better at directing patients and caregivers on how to be the provider's hands, become better at ensuring patients have the right technologies, and improve their "webside manner," otherwise known as telehealth etiquette. Finally, improved effectiveness also comes with taking the time to step back and develop clinical protocols.

Providers are not the only ones thinking long term. Movement at the policy level is also taking place. Many efforts are already underway to make temporary policy changes more permanent ones. A few challenging issues on the policy front that will need to be confronted include the following:

- Reimbursement for telephone (audio-only) services. We have to figure out that "sweet spot" where there is sufficient reimbursement for providers who must use telephone (audio-only) communications to ensure access to care for patients/clients without broadband or appropriate video-enabled devices, without creating a disincentive for using videoconference technologies when available.

- Privacy and security. Now that providers and patients have experienced the ease of connecting with each other using familiar consumer-based devices and platforms, moving to devices and/or platforms that are more secure may be more frustrating. Technology and platform vendors will need to be cognizant of the user experience.

- Lack of alignment between Medicare, Medicaid, and commercial payers. This will continue to be a frustration for practices desiring to offer telehealth to all patients. Aligning billing and coding protocols across all payor sources would greatly

simplify the process for providers and eliminate the barrier
of having to identify whether a telehealth service will be
covered before making it available to a patient.

- Inevitable "bad players." These are individuals or institutions
  who will raise questions and create greater scrutiny of telehealth due to activities related to fraud, waste, and abuse.

- Competition. Competition exists between small practices and
  "for-profit" companies and others who want to capitalize
  on the favorable policy environment and the newly gained
  receptivity to telehealth from patients.

- A barrage of legislation. Efforts to impact the telehealth policy
  landscape at state and federal levels ignited because of
  the pandemic. At the federal level, US representative Ann
  Wagner (R-MO) introduced HR 7992 (Telehealth Act) that
  combines nine telehealth bills into one piece of legislation. The legislation would provide various expansions in
  Medicare reimbursement for telehealth, including coverage
  for telemental health services without geographic and site
  restrictions, allowing FQHCs and RHCs to serve as distant
  site providers and more.

While COVID-19 continues to create societal challenges on
many fronts, every cloud has its silver lining. For those of us who
have been working for years to drive utilization of telehealth, we witnessed COVID-19 push forward the digital transformation of health
care by about a decade in less than a year. We have learned that telehealth can replace in-person visits for many visit types. Policies that
have not kept up with telehealth use or technologies have been a
historic barrier to widespread adoption of telehealth, and removing
those policy barriers became easier as the realities of the pandemic
made themselves manifest. Also, lack of broadband access is creating an infrastructure barrier to telehealth adoption, and care must
be taken to ensure that the growth of telehealth does not exacerbate
disparities in care.

Nevertheless, the "new normal" for health care will forever be changed to include telehealth technologies because of this pandemic.

## REFERENCES

1 Thielke, A., King, V. *Electronic Consultations (eConsults): A Triple Win for Patients, Clinicians, and Payers.* Milbank Memorial Fund, June 2020. https://www.milbank.org/wp-content/uploads/2020/06/eConsults_Milbank_Report_v4.pdf.

2 The Deloitte 2018 surveys of US health care consumers and physicians. Deloitte. https://www2.deloitte.com/xe/en/insights/industry/health-care/new-2018-surveys-US-health-care-consumers-physicians.html. Accessed August 30, 2022.

3 Nespor, C. A short history of stethoscopes. Melnick Medical Museum Blog, December 1, 2009. https://melnickmedicalmuseum.com/2009/12/01/a-short-history-of-stethoscopes.

4 Rangachari, P., Rissing, P., Rethemeyer, K. Awareness of evidence-based practices alone does not translate to implementation: insights from implementation research. *Quality Management in Health Care.* 2013;22(2):117–125. doi:10.1097/QMH.0b013e31828bc21d.

5 Buis, L., Singer, D., Solway, E., Kirch, M., Kullgren, J., Malani, P. Telehealth use among older adults before and during COVID-19. University of Michigan National Poll on Healthy Aging, August 17, 2020. http://hdl.handle.net/2027.42/156253.

# 4

---

## Bracing Early for a Delayed Impact

*How Appalachia's COVID-19 Timelines Affected*
*Health System Bottom Lines*

KATHY OSBORNE STILL

*Editor's Note: Rural zones across America saw different*
*outbreak patterns than urban ones. Appalachia's emotional*
*and economic depletion of human and capital resources*
*throughout the spring and summer of 2020 proved extensive.*
*Yet infection rates remained low in many rural localities,*
*raising the volume on public rumblings against restrictions*
*and precautions. Administrators throughout this "pandemic*
*midseason" calculated thankless math. Strategic moves to*
*minimize human danger put hospitals at greater risk of*
*closure long term and caused relationship difficulties in the*
*community. Then the school and holiday season began, the*
*virus really did show up, and everything got worse.*

A deadly global pandemic quickly filled the intensive care
units and critical care areas of the nation's hospitals. Health-
care workers were overburdened as they looked after droves of
COVID-19 patients while watching and silently worrying as their
supply of personal protective equipment (PPE) dwindled with no
true hope of replenishment in sight. The PPE that suppliers still had
in stock came with exploding prices that also placed a fiscal burden
on hospitals and hospital chains.

Just as it seemed the health-care situation could not worsen, hospital administrators clicked through the corporate spreadsheets and found that revenue, like the PPE supplies, had dried up. Elective surgeries were halted to accommodate anticipated and actual surges in COVID-19 cases, patients delayed preventive care visits, and some with chronic conditions feared contracting the virus more than the life-threatening issues they already faced. The emergency rooms still did a brisk business, but the health-care services that drew the biggest revenue—patients with generous health insurance cards—were just not enough to keep coffers full.

The American Hospital Association reported in early spring that the nation's hospitals would lose more than $320 million by the end of 2020, mostly due to the costs related to the pandemic and the loss of revenue that came with the public's fear of visiting physicians and hospitals in general.[1]

Layoffs and furloughs of employees, including nursing and other critical health-care positions, soon followed in late March and April. Physicians and some administrators, including senior staff, received pay cuts. The public was left wondering why such an illogical move would make sense, but hospital leaders said there was no choice. Cuts were needed to keep hospitals open, even during the pandemic.

The American Hospital Association also reported that about 270 hospitals issued furloughs just weeks after the virus spiked in the spring. The furloughed workers were eligible for unemployment benefits, and most kept their health insurance and other benefits. Across the nation, this varied widely.[1]

Hospitals in the Appalachian Mountain region were particularly vulnerable to the financial crisis COVID-19 brought. Ballad Health, a corporation that operates about 21 health-care facilities, mainly in northeastern Tennessee and southwestern Virginia, announced in early April that it would furlough 1,300 employees and would implement a 10 to 20 percent pay reduction for some physicians and administrators at the vice president rank. The furlough represented about 9 percent of the corporation's 15,000 workers. Ballad CEO Alan Levine said the COVID-19 crisis had put a severe strain on the organization.

"We are all experiencing the anxiety, stress and uncertainty this pandemic has unleashed," Levine said in a news release. "Businesses large and small, families, churches, schools, governments and health-care organizations are each struggling with the sudden and traumatic structural changes that have rocked our lives and our livelihoods."[2]

Levine said the organization took aggressive steps to increase its PPE supply and to keep its employees and the public updated on the ongoing situation. It wasn't just Ballad feeling the effects; many health-care systems that the virus had not reached by late April and May 2020 implemented a similar strategy. Citing the COVID crisis and the loss of elective surgeries, Pikeville Medical Center (PMC) in eastern Kentucky furloughed 200 in late April. "We are thankful that our government leaders have understood the necessity to support and financially assist hospitals and our most important asset, our dedicated staff members," said Donovan Blackburn, PMC CEO and vice president of the board of directors.

Blackburn said PMC had to protect its employees while being fiscally responsible, in order to sustain the hospital for future generations.[3] PMC said it planned to bring the workers back full-time within a few weeks, and it fulfilled its promise. As reported in September in *Becker's Hospital Review,* just over 25 workers were still awaiting a return to work.

The nation seemed to tire quickly of COVID-19 health and safety measures, even though spikes still popped up in various cities and rural areas. This sense of "denial well-being" on display as summer wore on caused an uptick in the fiscal situation for hospitals. Facilities called most furloughed workers back as hospitals and medical centers restarted nonemergency procedures, and physicians in clinics welcomed patients who returned to waiting rooms once again.

While infectious disease experts repeatedly warned that the next wave of COVID-19 was on the way or in some cases already here, hospital leaders worked quickly to harness the lessons learned from treating COVID-19 patients in the first six months, as well as those with other medical concerns during a pandemic. They moved from predictive behavior based on spiking short term to protecting the health and safety of patients and the hospitals' fiscal health at the same time and tried to incorporate safety protocols that allowed a return to electives and general care.

Then, as these experts and local hospital system leaders predicted, the wave arrived in the fall, and it was akin to a tsunami. Ballad Health frantically searched for 350 nurses to staff facilities in its 29-county service area. The system announced its staffing needs via Twitter, as social media became the chief communication venue in many cases. In weekly news conferences, Ballad officials sought the public's help by asking the entire community to wear masks and stay away from even small gatherings. Adding to the mix was the different way Virginia and Tennessee governors issued mask requirements and related health and safety measures. Virginia opted for a stricter stance, while Tennessee was a bit looser, allowing mayors and county executives to issue their own measures. Both were inside this single hospital system.

By November 5, Ballad was treating more than 190 COVID-19 patients in its 21 facilities. Of the overall number, 41 were in intensive care units (ICUs). The surge drastically increased after the Thanksgiving holiday, when many in the service area ignored public health and safety guidelines in favor of spending time with grandma—even though their decision put elderly relatives and those at high risk in peril.

Levine, the Ballad CEO, said in a December 3 news conference that misinformation and outright indifference were primarily to blame for the record-setting surge. "There are people by that bedside literally holding the hands of people who are dying, many of whom didn't even believe us when we told them they had COVID," Levine said.[4]

To drive that point home, Levine played a video of Emily N. Egan, an ICU nurse, as she discussed what she and her coworkers were coping with during the pandemic and the unprecedented local surge in cases. Her words were poignant, and her voice was strained with exhaustion and frustration. "We started this fight together," she began. "We started staying home and not going out unnecessarily. As a community, I think everybody did really well.

They fought with us trying to stop the spread. We felt like they were behind us."

Egan seemed defeated at times as she spoke about the change in the community's attitude. Her description of body bags was a swift and brutal gut punch.

"Now I guess you're tired of being alone or at home and want to get out and be social again," she said. "I understand the importance of mental health, but the fight is getting worse. It's spreading. We are losing more people than we are keeping. I've put an ungodly amount of people in body bags. We lost them."

She spoke of carrying the job home with her each day and how many tears she had shed in the process. "I understand sacrifice, but seeing these people die who can't breathe just starts to take a toll on you," she said. "I've sat with them and held their hands as they died."

Egan pleaded with the public to take the virus seriously and to take steps to stem the spread of COVID. She then went back to the ICU to care for her many patients.[5]

Levine called health-care workers such as Egan true heroes, and he stressed that they were in a struggle as the virus surge continued. "ICU nurses are not fragile people," he said. "They deal with a lot. Then to get in the car and hear people say they don't have to wear masks or eschewing the idea of social distancing. Not practicing proven steps to avoid the spread of the virus doesn't make you cool, it makes you dangerous."[4]

Ballad decided to again suspend elective surgeries for 30 days beginning on December 7, 2020. The hospital system chose to reassign staff to help combat the surge, which conformed to the prediction that it would double by the end of December. Balance sheets balanced against community needs proved financially costly to the hospital system.

In yet another news conference, Ballad leaders said the rapid increase in COVID-19 patients was a primary reason to halt nonemergency surgeries. Levine said there would be no employee furloughs that December, unlike the first time elective surgeries were stopped during the spring portion of the pandemic. Instead, it was all hands to the COVID surge. "We're obviously very concerned about the capacity issue, but we've got to be proactive and move to redeploy staff as opposed to having it hit our front door and not be prepared for it," Levine told news crews and the public, who were viewing the press conference via social media.

Utilizing the National Guard to work at some COVID-19 testing centers also helped staffing shortages, by freeing up some nurses and other clinical workers to care for patients rather than conducting tests. Ballad officials did not provide specifics but spoke of having plans to create more staffing options if the situation grew dire.

As bed capacity was nearly at 94 percent and ICU beds were at 92 percent in early December, Ballad announced it had rented refrigerated mobile morgues to prepare for the crisis in caseloads that was anticipated to arrive shortly before Christmas. Some in the public took to social media and railed against scare tactics, as the health system displayed photographs of the mobile morgue trucks. Some questioned whether the trucks were actually refrigerated units. These comments were likely on Levine's mind at yet another December press conference, as he speculated that partisan politics and a misinformation campaign were troubling. "There are two things Ballad Health can do in this," he said. "One is to be the best caregivers we can be, and No. 2 is we can try to be a constant source of truth throughout this crisis. There is nothing more important than information and nothing more damaging than misinformation."[4]

Levine also cited hospital statistics that one in six COVID-19 patients who entered the ICU would die there. A nurse like Egan should be holding their hand when they do, but the unspoken coda was that Ballad was running out of staff to provide such humanitarian moments.

Nearby, Pikeville Medical Center added a new floor to care for COVID-19 patients. The move came in early November, as eastern Kentucky coped with its own surge. PMC now had two units dedicated to COVID-19 patients. The new center came as PMC treated its 700th COVID patient. The unit received three more patients in its new 32-bed unit on the first day.

As with Ballad, PMC said it was looking at other ways to expand the COVID units and to find enough staff to help care for the patients as the surge exploded. Blackburn echoed the same concerns about misinformation as officials as Ballad expressed. The public must understand that the situation is dire and that all must do their part to combat the pandemic and the swath of devastation that was sweeping eastern Kentucky. A lack of open ICU beds was a looming issue, but staffing was also a major concern. A surge in cases, Blackburn said, would result in employees stretched by longer hours and a subsequent higher risk of contracting the virus—with exponentially disastrous consequences to staffing. "We're not testing more, we're testing about equal, we're seeing our positive rates go up and we're seeing our hospitalizations go up substantially, and it's putting a lot of pressure on organizations like us," he said.

It is not an easy task to open a new ICU unit because of the stringent regulations and a lengthy approval process. However, the need for qualified health-care workers, especially when those skilled workers are in high demand during the pandemic, is a troublesome concern. "An ICU room is designed . . . to be an ICU," Blackburn said. "We also have to go through a process to be able to be accredited and actually licensed to be able to have an ICU."

As for skilled health-care workers, Blackburn stressed that nurses have different skill sets and specialties. The same goes for physicians. "The ability to have staff and to be able to staff up just doesn't exist to go from x-amount to x-amount," he said. "We're seeing this huge demand for nursing staff throughout the country, not just nursing staff but providers as well, because you also have to have a physician in order to house more patients."[6]

Health system and hospital administrators agreed that protecting employees is vital. To do otherwise would decrease the number of skilled workers needed to care for patients in all communities. The frontline health-care workers are more important than ever as the nation copes with the fallout of the global pandemic. It's all about the people, the health system leaders agreed. The capacity issue no longer rested with beds and ventilators but with staff to run them.

Yet the economic issues will persist, for rural hospitals in massive ways but for all hospitals in some ways. Furloughs ending sounds like a good thing, but when the revenue-generating surgeries that keep most hospitals ticking along are set aside in order to deal with a tsunami of viral cases, the hospital will face long-term financial issues. This makes Levine's remarks about misinformation particularly ironic—or perhaps poignant. In pointing out that hospitals do not have a financial incentive to overreport COVID-19 cases, or even to seek to take more cases than other hospitals, Levine has put his finger on something that hospital leaders nationwide fear to touch. Discussing financial health with more than 400,000 dead before the vaccines arrived was unseemly and politically inexpedient. Yet the topic had to be addressed: treating large numbers of COVID-19 patients doesn't benefit hospitals financially; in fact, it harms them.

Rural hospitals will take years to climb out of the financial holes into which the virus has thrown them.

Couple the rampant disinformation activity on social media regarding masks and distancing measures and the exhaustion of the public for staying home with this economic hot potato, and it is hard to tell which will be most damaging in the long run.

### REFERENCES

1 AHA report: Hospital financial losses from COVID-19 expected to top $323 billion in 2020. American Hospital Association, June 30, 2022. https://www.aha.org/news/headline/2020-06-30-aha-report-hospital-financial-losses-covid-19-expected-top-323-billion.
2 Ballad Health announces added investment for nursing, direct care team to ensure availability during possible COVID-19 surge. Ballad Health, April 8, 2020. https://www.balladhealth.org/news/announces-investment-employee-assistance.
3 Pikeville Medical Center announces furlough plans. *Appalachian News-Express,* April 24, 2020. https://news-expressky.com/covid-19/pikeville-medical-center-announces-furlough-plans/article_4a9c2a60-8676-11ea-9940-b3338005f9d2.html.
4 McGee, D. Misinformation, indifference fuels local COVID-19 spike. *Bristol Herald Courier,* December 4, 2020.

5 Ballad Health Facebook page. Emily Nichole Egan, RN, has been at Ballad Health for 8 years. She's an experienced ICU nurse who is now serving in our COVID-19 unit at Holston Valley Medical Center. Please listen to Emily's story about what life is currently like for our #healthcareheroes. #balladhealth. December 2, 2020. https://www.facebook.com/watch/?v=2469298246708828. Accessed August 31, 2022.

6 Ziege, N. "Focus on the facts": PMC CEO warns public to "wake up" after continuous spike in COVID-19 hospitalizations. *Appalachian News-Express,* November 13, 2020. https://news-expressky.com/news/focus-on-the-facts-pmc-ceo-warns-public-to-wake-up-after-continuous-spike-in/article_2143bf22-2598-11eb-8284-dfae5cb88575.html.

**Part 2**

---

# STORIES

# 5

## Passover

LYNN ELLIOTT

*Editor's Note: With the preceding backgrounds informing the big picture, we now enter storytelling mode. Elliott offers the human face of health-care workers awaiting central Appalachia's delayed surge. Her story compliments Still's economics explanation and LeBoeuf's account of logistical challenges facing those who train the future doctors of Appalachia.*

Becoming a physician is daunting under normal circumstances, where work schedules are capped at 80 hours a week and residents typically have just four days off every month. In addition, young doctors are expected to read up on the discipline they are rotating in that month. A rotation at the children's hospital for family medicine residents means working alongside residents who are specifically training in pediatrics and the accompanying expectation to be equally knowledgeable. A rotation in gastroenterology requires advance reading in six areas of the most common gastrointestinal (GI) diseases. Preparing for board certification in a medical specialty means not just being familiar with dozens of areas of medicine, like endocrinology and neurology, but mastering that material by being able to diagnose and treat patients with those conditions.

Throw in a pandemic, and one might expect these doctors in training to crack under the mental pressure. In an amazing display of fortitude that makes me even more proud of them than I usually am, the residents in our hospital shouldered all the additional pressure of COVID-19, put on their masks, and kept going.

For months after March 2020, when the nation shut down and cases exploded in urban centers like New York City and Seattle, COVID-19 was mostly hypothetical in southwestern Virginia. Stories on the news about hospitals overrun with patients were in big cities, places we in our small Appalachian town were accustomed to see go crazy from time to time with various trends or problems that rarely affected us. The pandemic was supposed to be different, a literal global health threat from which no one, not even us, tucked up in our cozy corner, was safe.

The hospital where I work with residents who are training for medical practice in family medicine and internal medicine prepared for a storm of patients that didn't materialize—not in April, nor across the summer of 2020, nor well into fall. Waiting for the wave to hit became exhausting.

Living in a rural area did for a time seem to help the odds of avoiding COVID. Rural life means people can walk their dogs down Main Street and not pass another person. Some remained cavalier enough to go to the grocery store without wearing a mask. Those of us who wore them thought those who didn't were foolish, and I suspect those without masks thought the same of us.

It wasn't just urban disdain, though. My region is the buckle of the Bible Belt, so lots of messages by locals on social media asserted that God is in control. People encouraged one another to believe the angel of death would pass over them. A man I know told me proudly, midsummer 2020, that he had shaken hands three times the day before. When I asked how he could do that when he has children at home, he replied that his faith teaches him to "be not afraid." (I guess that means fear isn't the reason so many people have guns in my part of the country.)

In anticipation of an onslaught of patients, the hospital system announced there would be furloughs, which took place on the Jewish holiday of Passover. Knowing that wave was coming felt like waiting for a root canal without Novocain. Before it hit, more than

10 percent of the workforce was put on a 90-day furlough. In my department of graduate medical education, the angel of employment death did pass over us (despite no one scribbling over the office door with a red Sharpie; for those unfamiliar, in the biblical book of Exodus 12:1–29, those who put blood on their door frames were passed over by the angel of death).

Although our health-care system needed to save money to stay afloat and be ready to serve when that ever-predicted tsunami of patients arrived, everyone knew that reducing the number of doctors we were training to serve in rural Appalachia would be suicidal. More than ever, we needed them to be ready. Hence, my department was spared.

There was no public announcement of who was furloughed and who was not, just an out-of-office reply to an email revealing someone wasn't at work. Sometimes a name came up in casual conversation of a colleague who was furloughed—although I must add that casual conversations were few and far between in our tense hospital halls. COVID, furloughs, and masks made it exhausting to converse for anything other than official business. Each time we realized someone wasn't there, it reinforced a sobering realization that, like contracting COVID-19, it could have happened to any of us.

It wasn't just the hospital staff who were affected by this constant message of "it's coming, it's coming." Some locals—a minority, perhaps, yet a vocal one—began to express on social media that Appalachian health-care administrators were crying wolf. When the virus failed to take hold here in the ways people heard about on the national news in places like Dallas and Miami, locals became less patient about the restrictions; some even translated the peace of our region into belief that national news had faked the seriousness of the crisis in other places.

It is stressful to come to the hospital, even when you're not a patient. It's important to remember that those who work in a hospital see people on what can be the worst day of their lives. They seldom know whether they should be in the main hospital or the outpatient building or how to get where they need to go. Even without the stress of a pandemic, they don't know the rules and are easily frustrated by questions. The intense concentration on their faces indicates they will remember every single interaction. Being in the position of having information, and therefore power, can make it easy to forget how defenseless patients are. In every interaction, we have one chance to get it right.

That was exponentially evident during COVID-19. Compassion, compassion, compassion: we have to remember that, no matter how frightened we are, these patients are more afraid. We remain polite as we explain that they must wear masks and kind as we express regret that a loved one cannot accompany them. It strains and it drains us, but it is harder for them. I was proud of my colleagues for the compassion I saw them exhibit as summer dragged on.

Fall arrived, and with it came the wave; normally, anticipation giving way to reality would be celebrated, but not in this situation. The monster seeped through nursing homes first, and we snapped to attention. The first warning shots had been fired. And then the COVID patients just kept coming, and if we thought October was accelerating, we had not yet begun to understand how fast and how far this virus would burn through our area. The holidays loomed, and administrators told us to brace for impact again.

Broadly speaking, Appalachians have no greater or more sincerely held values than God and family. The holidays, celebrating both, were on our doorstep. We were already in a spike. Tempting as it might have been to retort, "You said that last time," we understood that the next wave would not only be on a more predicted schedule—within a week of Thanksgiving Day—but worse. Appalachians, like the rest of Americans, were exhausted. They wanted to see their families on Christmas and honor one of the two most important days on the Christian calendar. Perhaps the false sense of security throughout summer lulled some away from precautions. So many factors fed into what happened.

It has often occurred to me, working in a hospital, that you can see something coming, yet you can't get out of its way. All you can do is prepare for its arrival. This, too, is mentally exhausting.

Staff were recalled, surgeries postponed once again. Perhaps we hadn't been spared, but being late to the party did mean we could stock up on personal protective equipment, brush up on infection protocols, and preach social distancing and handwashing to patients before it was too late.

Post-Thanksgiving COVID cases soared; testing positivity rates (which in the early stages of the wave hovered around 10 percent) edged past 28 percent. Some of the residents said later that they resigned themselves to contracting COVID-19 that winter. Some did, despite all our precautions. Sheer volume made it inevitable.

Although the risk for contracting COVID was 12 times higher for health-care workers, it still felt like a coin toss as to who would get it—young versus old, cautious versus cavalier—that a roll of the dice seemed to decide who the invisible monster would weasel itself into and who it left alone.[1] When I say "cavalier," I don't mean brazenly uncompliant; a practitioner might adhere to all precautions and still contract COVID-19 by doing something unconsciously foolish like rubbing their tired eyes before washing their hands.

Two years into the pandemic, COVID-19 still weighed on the doctors in my residency program like a heavy blanket. The masks that were sweatboxes in summer became scratchy and uncomfortable in the winter. People were cranky and the refrain was that it will be nice when it ends; when vaccination began in the United Kingdom, we were glued to the news, waiting for an American announcement. Applause resounded when our vaccinations began. A different type of noise followed as we realized how many patients in our region were averse to getting a COVID vaccination.

I reminded myself that Anne Frank endured worse, and I stayed home as much as possible, even postvaccination. The joy of socializing with vaccinated friends and colleagues remains tempered with awareness of variants, viral loads, and other questions. It is not a great burden, given what's at stake. Being in close quarters is familiar to me. I lived in New York for five years, first in Brooklyn in a 500-square-foot apartment where our daughter was born. A year later we moved to the Upper West Side to a 702-square-foot apartment. It felt palatial—even though I'm sure the square footage included the closet. I can't imagine what it would be like to live in New York City now with a young child in a tiny box of an apartment whose floors sagged in the middle. Had my life taken a few different turns than those that brought me here, I could have been in that city dealing with the fear, uncertainty, and claustrophobia of this pandemic in an urban area.

Way back in March 2020, hospital administrators began staffing a screening desk to make sure patients and visitors didn't enter the hospital with a fever or other telltale symptoms. When visitors stopped being allowed inside, most were understanding; they realized that it was for everyone's safety and complied. Elderly patients had the hardest time with these new rules. One older man who couldn't hear well kept walking closer to me until I finally put my arm straight in front of me to keep him from being in my face. He wasn't being obstreperous; he just couldn't believe the world had changed that much and caught him up in it, and he didn't understand my mask-muffled instructions to stand still.

Most days I took the stairs to my office on the fourth floor to avoid contact with people in elevators. Trying to conserve masks, I wore the same one for a week at a time because I didn't have clinical contact with patients. One summer day, after reaching the fourth floor, I walked out of the stairwell breathing hard—just as a linen bin was being wheeled from the COVID unit. Maybe the elevator would have been safer.

Being conscious of disinfecting seemed like playing a game of cat and mouse. Before we knew the virus was mostly airborne, I would wipe down the laptops the residents use and consider them clean until someone touched one of them. Picking up my laundry from the hamper to take to the washer one night, I realized the clothes hugged to my chest were the ones I wore to work—so they had just potentially infected the clean pajamas I was wearing. I decided to spray Lysol on my pajama shirt and call it good.

We were all tired but knew it would take just one mistake to undo all the vigilance and effort to avoid infection. With vaccination,

many things changed for the better. I remember thinking prevac-
cination that every day I woke up feeling well confirmed that, as
of two weeks prior, I had not come in contact with the virus. The
13 days in between were a wild card.

I remember April 2020, when many parts of the country were
being slammed with COVID-19. On the night of April 6, the International Space Station glided across the sky of southwestern Virginia
like a small star. It was almost unimaginable to think there were humans encased in that little dot of light. From the astronauts' view, it
was probably equally unthinkable that so much suffering was happening on the beautiful blue marble outside their windows. Some 43,438
Americans learned they had COVID-19 and nearly 9,000 died from
the disease that day. By December 2020, those rates were exponentially
higher. That summer we spent bracing, we had no idea how long and
how hard the hit would be when it came. That pinprick of light gliding
above us seemed to me a symbol of hope, despair, and uncertainty all
at the same time. What an odd symbol it was—for an odd time.

Every June, I meet with new residents during orientation and
go over general information about the training program, like how to
report a safety issue and the protocol for dealing with a complaint.
June 2020 was unique because of COVID-19, but also because my
daughter started her residency in another part of the country. More
than ever, I wondered what the new residents were thinking about
as they prepared for training. Having a child start residency training during a pandemic is not what any parent would choose. My
impulse to remind her to eat well was replaced with wanting to drill
into her the steps for putting on and taking off personal protective
equipment in ways that avoid contamination.

As I talked with the residents at our program during orientation, I made a point to tell them they would want to run to every
code blue when a patient is dying and they would have to take the
time to put on the protective equipment. I told them, then, that it
was projected that 200,000 Americans were expected to die from
COVID-19 by October and to please not be one of them. How small
that number seems now!

Back in my office after that talk, I trusted that, in her residency so far from home, someone else was telling my daughter the same thing. I hoped that, like the space station, the angel of death would pass over us and that if the predicted tsunami was inevitable, then these residents, the future physicians of Appalachia, would defeat the angel bringing that wave of death and sadness with both science and compassion.

REFERENCE

1 Marquedant, K. Study reveals the risk of COVID-19 infection among health care workers. Massachusetts General Hospital, May 5, 2020. https://www.massgeneral.org/news/coronavirus/study-reveals-risk -of-covid-19-infection-among-health-care-workers.

# 6

---

# Working in the Hospital in the Early Days of the Pandemic

## LUCAS AIDUKAITIS

*Editor's Note: When the pandemic began, medical residents around the globe experienced exhilaration intermingled with panic. Training during a global health crisis: What could be better preparation? Slowly, realization set in that the virus would disrupt educational opportunity more than enhance it. And that doctors who knew how to protect themselves could still get sick.*

The coronavirus pandemic changed the world, and its effects are more than illness in the body. They include economic problems, social isolation, and loss of life. People of all walks of life suffered and still suffer, and none escape it, from the old to the young, the rich and poor.

By the time we had lived with this pandemic for a year, nearly everyone on the planet could spell *COVID* and *quarantine* backwards in their sleep. And yet, there was still so much that we did not know. Arguments continued in scientific research and among the general public: What was the best medical treatment for the virus? How deadly was the virus? What was the role of masks in preventing transmission of the disease?

Anywhere in the world at that time, you would find drastic changes caused directly or indirectly by the pandemic. Parks and roads once full of individuals walking and playing outside featured warning signs strongly recommending masks; restaurants and bars once packed with customers exclusively offered delivery or pickup services; religious services of all types of faiths carried their worship online or used socially distant choreography when in person. Schools, hospitals, sports, and nature itself felt the effects of the virus. Who could believe that the waters of Venice, Italy, would again feature dolphins?

In 1918, in the time of the deadly pandemic of influenza (often called the "Spanish flu"), many people recorded their experiences with the pandemic, much as we do today. Most of those stories stayed hidden until a descendant or historian found them in some dusty old family journal. In the twenty-first century, however, almost anyone affected by the current pandemic can have their story shared worldwide instantly on any number of electronic and physical media. We get to experience, therefore, a worldwide pandemic seasoned with the cultural customs of our home countries and hometowns.

To illustrate how important it is to broaden our experiences with a worldwide view, let us consider another momentous occasion celebrated in 2019: the 50th anniversary of the Apollo 11 moon landing. Consider Neil Armstrong and Buzz Aldrin, the astronauts on that flight who took the first and second steps on the Moon, respectively. They trained together, ate together, spoke to reporters and journalists together, and quarantined together both before and after their historic journey, and they struggled together to land the Lunar Module at Tranquility Base on the surface of the moon. How much would we have lost if one of them had decided not to write or talk about the journey and those first steps with the justification that their experiences were too similar and hence uninteresting? Armstrong famously said, "That's one small step for a man, one giant leap for mankind" when stepping onto the surface for the first time. Aldrin, upon seeing the lunar landscape, said instead, "Beautiful view. Magnificent desolation."

And what of Michael Collins, the third astronaut of Apollo 11 who went through much of the same training, traveling nearly all the way to the Moon only to have to stay orbiting around it while his two companions were making footprints in the lunar soil? In his terrific book *Carrying the Fire,* Collins records his feelings about the moment he was left alone around the moon: "I am alone now, truly alone, and absolutely isolated from any known life. I am it. If a count were taken, the score would be three billion plus two on the other side of the Moon, and one plus God knows what is on this side."[1] Is his story less "valuable" because he didn't land on the ultimate destination? Every story counts, and each new perspective contributes to understanding how COVID affected us individually and as a community. And here is mine, a small blip in the vast published and unpublished world.

I am a resident physician at a rural hospital located in the charming and historic city of Abingdon, Virginia, in central Appalachia, part of an integrated health system serving 29 counties of northeastern Tennessee, southwestern Virginia, northwestern North Carolina, and southeastern Kentucky. I also work at the Primary Care Center, an outpatient clinic that not only provides medical care to children and adults but also trains the next generation of doctors.

I graduated from medical school in 2019 from Liberty University College of Osteopathic Medicine in Lynchburg, Virginia, and prior to that, in 2013, I earned a BS in biochemistry from Brigham Young University in Provo, Utah. I was raised in Brazil and have numerous relatives living there and a number of others living in other countries, including the USA, Chile, Argentina, Portugal, Germany, Lithuania, and Luxemburg. We have kept in contact throughout this pandemic via emails and messaging apps, and fortunately no one in my immediate family has passed away from COVID—although at least half a dozen contracted the disease and recovered.

As a resident physician, I am employed by the hospital training me for three years before I can practice medicine independently. Every four weeks, my 14 fellow family medicine residents and I rotate to a different hospital service as part of our training. These include pediatrics, hospital medicine, clinic, night shift, cardiology, gastroenterology, critical care, psychiatry, and a number of electives for us to choose from, like wound care, neurology, geriatrics, sports medicine, and others. In conjunction with our rotations, each of us also has a panel of patients that we care for at the Primary Care Clinic.

Before coronavirus became a household name, an email was sent to the medical staff on January 9, 2020, from Dr. Peters, the chief medical officer of our hospital, informing us of a focus on "pneumonia of unknown etiology" from Wuhan, China. The email stated that the illness was evolving, that no cases had yet been detected outside of China, and that symptoms appeared to involve coughing and shortness of breath for the majority, but a few developed serious respiratory problems. At that time there was also no data proving that human-to-human transmission was happening.

Whenever an email like this is received, I take a minute to consider the likelihood of the illness becoming something we will have to screen our patients for. A similar email was sent months before informing us of an outbreak of hepatitis A in our region of Appalachia. My colleagues and I knew right away that the hepatitis A outbreak was very relevant to us, so we got to work. We advocated for hepatitis A testing for our patients, handwashing prior to eating or touching one's face, and vaccinating for hepatitis A if patients enjoyed eating out. And as acute hepatitis A cases became less common in our hospital and clinic, we shifted focus to other local health concerns.

Would this "pneumonia of unknown etiology" become relevant? It certainly didn't seem likely to do so in January of 2020. I could not imagine any of my patients spending any time in Wuhan, China; our region is very far away from international airports, and it just seemed far fetched at the time to even worry about an illness that had no confirmed mode of transmission in a land very far away. Even if it eventually left China, the likelihood of it affecting Appalachia appeared very low.

January 2020 proceeded as usual. I had just finished a busy month in my general surgery rotation, where our hospital census (the number of patients assigned to the surgical team in the hospital) fluctuated between 15 and 25 patients per day. I was happy for the learning, yet excited for a change of pace in my next rotation—but the change of pace never came. We had just as many patients with the cardiology group as we did in surgery. I reminded myself that being busy is not a bad thing; how can a doctor or nurse or student learn how to treat patients if they don't see many patients in a day? The data of admitted patients to our hospital shows that the hospital census remained relatively high from the end of 2019 to the end of February. From a maximum of 115 staffed hospital beds available, the weekly average number of patients in the hospital was about 73 per day, with a low of 66 and a high of 102 in that period. This includes all patients in the intensive care unit (ICU), progressive care unit, labor and delivery unit, and regular hospital floor. Add to the daily hospital and clinic work the interminable political bickering on TV and radio, endless sports to stream on the internet and watch in person, and movies and theater productions to enjoy outside the home, and you have a typical picture of what life was like for several of us prepandemic in this part of the planet.

Then February 2020 came along, and news about COVID-19 (as it was now starting to be called) became more frequent. The virus invaded Italy and other European nations; it had spread to Africa and South America, albeit in lesser numbers; and it was continuing to devastate Wuhan. A follow-up email from Dr. Peters updated us on the status of the virus: it had finally been confirmed to transmit through human-to-human contact. At this time, there were no confirmed cases in most of central Appalachia, although some people were in quarantine despite testing negative for COVID.

This is the moment that subtle changes began at the hospital. During one of my mornings doing rounds with patients as part of the cardiology team, we found an area on the fourth floor that typically sees patients only for observation, and overnight stays had been isolated with movable walls and yellow tape, with a single entrance on one side to minimize unnecessary entry and exit to that part of the hospital. My initial thought was "This seems excessive," but the thought was fleeting and we moved on to find another way to see our patient.

However, news of the spread of the virus became ever more common in the media. By mid-February we learned that almost

50,000 patients had been infected in China, 2,000 of them health-care workers. The United States had 15 cases. Many religious services were changed from in-person service to online only, and many sport competitions were canceled outright.

When March came around, I was assigned to work in the emergency room (ER). I recall coming in at around 1 p.m. on my first day and seeing all 28 ER beds occupied and another 20 patients sitting in the waiting room waiting for their turn to be evaluated. Understandably, I got a very brief orientation and was put to work straightaway. A critical skill you learn in the ER is that you need to lay eyes on a patient very quickly and make a decision based on their main complaint and vital signs as to whether they need immediate medical attention. "Chest pain" and "shortness of breath" are very common concerns that patients come to the hospital for, and these must be looked at very quickly, as one can die in minutes from a heart attack (which commonly causes both symptoms); at the same time, many complaints of "chest pain" or "shortness of breath" have little or nothing to do with the heart—or even the lungs. Anxiety, for example, won't kill you immediately, but it can make you breathless or cause chest pain. You will never know unless you see the patient first, and you can't assume.

On that first day, I saw 11 patients; as fast as we could see them and either admit to the hospital or send them back home, another patient would take their place, and we would evaluate, treat, admit, or send the patient back home. This wasn't the pandemic yet; it was a typical day in the ER before COVID-19, full of people seeking care for their health.

The ER has a different census from that of the hospital. Many patients coming to the emergency department don't end up getting admitted to the hospital, and this is by design. The ER stabilizes critically ill patients and admits those that need more time for stabilization prior to returning home. If a patient is not critically ill and comes to the ER, chances are they will be observed for some time, then be discharged home; a few of these patients are admitted and cared for in the hospital for a variety of reasons: their illness is not critical but their social situation is dangerous (think patients at risk for abuse or in unsafe living situations); or their illness is not currently critical but has the potential for deterioration quickly (think chronic obstructive lung disease or congestive heart failure, where small changes in blood volume or mild infection can suddenly overwhelm the body's delicate balance).

Many of these decisions are made with the input of the patient, ER physician, hospital admitting physician, and others involved in their care, like parents, children, and other family members. People coming to the ER do so for a variety of reasons, and it can be a gauge for how the community perceives the seriousness of an illness juxtaposed against what is happening with the world at large. I recall, for instance, a very empty ER during the Monster Energy NASCAR Cup Series on August 19, 2019, and a very full ER the following day. It was apparent to me at the time that going to the ER could wait until the local NASCAR race—and subsequent celebration—was over.

During the first two weeks of March of 2020, when COVID-19 was ramping up in the United States, the ER was full as it usually was. A daily average of 88 patients came to the emergency department from March 1 to 16, with a low of 82 and a high of 103. I would see an average of 10 patients per 12-hour shift and feel very exhausted by the end of it. I had a particularly busy day on March 13, with many patients being evaluated for chest pain and shortness of breath, and I was grateful at getting a few days break before having to come back to work on March 18.

When I returned that day, I found a very different emergency room. Instead of seeing 12 patients, I only saw 7. The average number of patients coming to the emergency department fell from an average of 80 to 48 almost overnight. March 19 saw our last peak of patients at 87, and on March 20 we saw only 54 all day. The number of patients coming to be seen in the emergency room reached a historic low of 33 on April 2. It was not until April 27 that the numbers rebounded, with 69 patients evaluated. It was as if all of southwestern Appalachia decided at the same time that it was better to stay home than to risk getting exposed to a novel illness in the hospital waiting room.

As the coronavirus situation continued to evolve in the United States, the doctors in the emergency department talked about what was coming and how to prepare for it. It was fascinating to hear their arguments for and against certain decisions. For example, one argued that the emergency department should screen people prior to entering the emergency room and send them away if they were suspected to have COVID but were otherwise healthy. The positive side of screening at that point would be to minimize the number of people sitting in the waiting room to whom an individual with COVID could transmit the virus. One doctor then replied that such a policy, while possibly preventing hospital transmission of the disease, would likely violate the Emergency Medical Treatment and Active Labor Act (EMTALA) laws. EMTALA was passed in 1986 in the United States to protect individuals from hospitals turning them away for failure to carry insurance or for their anticipated inability to pay the high cost of care. It also protects patients from coming to the emergency room and being turned away by a physician who is too tired or annoyed to examine the patient. Any human who walks into an American hospital campus with an emergency room is entitled by law to a medical screening exam to evaluate if an emergency medical condition exists. If it does, the hospital must provide care for that condition or transfer the patient to a hospital that can care for him or her. The receiving hospital must also accept that patient regardless of whether they have insurance.

So in the case of COVID-19, an interesting problem arose: EMTALA requires everyone seeking care to be examined, which would inevitably lead to a queue somewhere inside a closed room—perfect for a virus that spreads between people in close contact. A simple solution would be to prescreen those with "COVID-like" symptoms (fever, cough, shortness of breath) and tell them to go home and call their doctor for a COVID test. But what if they were very short of breath? What if we sent these people home and they died on their way? By sending people home without a screening exam, were we violating EMTALA? Also, who would provide the screening? Would it be an ER doctor? Would it be a nurse? Would it be a receptionist?

The debate continued for several days until eventually it was decided that people should come to the emergency department if they felt they needed to be medically screened. At the same time, radio announcements, emails, and public announcements on news channels instructed patients who believed they were sick but not seriously so with COVID-19 to call a 24-7 nursing hotline dedicated to COVID screening and then follow the instructions for receiving additional medical care. It was a good compromise and effective use of technology to reach out to many people and minimize exposure in the hospital setting. Four rooms in the emergency department were designated "COVID rooms," equipped with personal protective equipment, and not used unless the patients were COVID confirmed or COVID suspected, to further isolate suspected cases from other providers and patients.

When I was not on ER duty, my wife and I took the opportunity to purchase staple foods (white rice and black beans, pasta, and fruit cans) in case we could not leave the house. It was a very stressful and anxious time that only got worse when, seven days later, schools throughout the state of Virginia were first suspended for two weeks and then outright canceled. We had to adjust quickly to this new reality of having a very early—and very long—summer ahead of us. Social mingling was out; social isolation became the norm. At least we were lucky enough to get a piano from a friend from church in the final days of pre-COVID normality.

Toward the end of March 2020, I no longer entered my home through the front door. Instead, I would go through the basement garage door, thoroughly shower in the laundry room, put my hospital clothes in the washer, don fresh clothes that had not been in the hospital, and then make my way upstairs to greet the family after a long day. It took me almost a full month before I no longer found this odd. It had become part of my daily routine, just another step I had to take to stay healthy and protect my family, like washing my hands and using hand sanitizer.

After a rare weekend that I was able to enjoy at home without work, I returned to the emergency room expecting another day running around trying my best to help patients. I found that the hospital was making additional changes to adapt to the incoming virus.

Hospital administration elected to make further rooms in the hospital available for COVID patients only. These rooms needed to be fitted with negative pressure devices to keep the air from circulating into the general hospital. All of the fourth floor, most of the third, and some of the second floor were closed off in preparation for the patient surge we were expecting. Elective surgeries were canceled; only emergency surgeries could be performed. Medical offices in the hospital began an intensive adjustment to phone and video consultations in lieu of face-to-face office visits whenever possible. Later it would also be decided that no visitors were allowed to enter the hospital except in some very specific situations (such as births, deaths, and end-of-life care).

The cafeteria closed its buffet services and replaced the salad bar with prepackaged salads and sandwiches. All tables for sitting were pushed to the side to minimize close contact with others. Outside dining was also closed to everyone, and entry to the hospital was allowed only in front of the emergency department and behind the hospital where ambulances drop off patients. All employees were required to use face masks when seeing patients, and efficient N95 respirators were distributed to those who would be most exposed to confirmed and suspected COVID patients. These face masks were initially in short supply, so we were instructed to disinfect them by leaving them exposed to the sun and replace them only once the masks became visibly soiled with dirt or sweat.

These changes appeared dramatic and over the top to some, and in hindsight they may even have been so, since the virus did not follow urban patterns in our rural area, and the anticipated peak in cases came only many months after these changes were implemented, but we knew no better and needed to prepare for the worst. As a fellow resident eloquently remarked, "Before 'problems' hit the fan, every preparation will seem excessive; but after it does, nothing that will be done thereafter will be enough." We had no way of knowing at the time the true extent and exposure our area would get to the novel coronavirus. We had to do our part to prepare for the worst.

Nevertheless, some of these decisions did have unintended consequences. For example, one problem we faced was this drastic drop in patients coming to the hospital. Hospitals employ a lot of people, from the obvious (nurses, doctors, phlebotomists) to less obvious (security guards, cafeteria employees, including cooks and servers for all the patients, case managers to help transition the patients safely from the hospital to home or elsewhere, among many others). All of these people play a crucial role in the proper and effective functioning of the hospital, and all need to receive wages to care for themselves and their families. Hospitals can't employ a full staff without a full census; otherwise they run the risk of not being capable of paying all these employees. When people were screened out of the emergency room when presenting with a cough and sneeze, the hospital saw fewer people admitted. Furthermore, the cancellation of needed but elective surgeries like screening colonoscopies and cardiac stress tests and cholecystectomies reduced even more the number of patients being admitted for care. Suddenly the number of providers and employees greatly outnumbered the number of patients in the hospital census. Consequently, almost every doctor took a pay cut; many nurses and midlevel providers were furloughed. Other employees were fired.

Residents like myself were more fortunate. Our jobs are secured as part of our contract to receive training in a teaching hospital. Hospitals receive a payment for every resident in their service, so cutting our work down more would only worsen things for the hospital; it would lose this source of income as well as have fewer people to cover those patients in the hospital. But we also suffered, albeit in a different way.

Our training requires us to see patients in the attached clinic as well as in the hospital. A decision was made early in March to split all residents between two groups: one group solely responsible for patients in the clinic, the other solely responsible for patients in the hospital. Occasionally, residents assigned to the hospital could see clinic patients over the phone, but this was limited to the more seasoned residents. The idea was to minimize cross-contamination between a resident being exposed to COVID in the hospital and then going to the clinic and exposing their patients and the rest of the staff, and vice-versa.

I have a number of patients who are Spanish-speaking only, and as a fluent Spanish provider I was expecting to be assigned to the clinic to care for this special-needs population, but I was instead assigned to work in the hospital for the next several months. My patients had to be rescheduled with other providers through an interpreter to get the care that they needed, while others had their appointments bumped forward several months. Several missed out on timely vaccinations such as pertussis, tetanus, diphtheria, *Haemophilus influenzae,* and pneumococcal shots, which protect infants from deadly diseases like pneumonia and meningitis. These patients eventually found a Spanish-speaking provider who was available to care for them, but for many months they struggled to get the care they needed for themselves and their children.

In the name of preventing the spread of COVID, many clinics unfortunately closed certain doors to patient health that in 2019 would have been available for them to use, doors like "same-day-office" appointments for new patients, in-person appointments for acute medical problems, and face-to-face counseling for patients struggling with anxiety, depression, and other psychological and psychiatric conditions. These patients could find care only one way: through the emergency room. The following examples help illustrate this point.

One patient in her mid-40s came to the emergency room with complaints of fatigue. There was no complaint of the triad "cough, fever, shortness of breath" we used at the time to screen for COVID-19, so I was given the green light to go examine her. She explained that she was feeling exhausted after exerting minimal effort over the last two months, despite not doing anything particularly different during that same period. She would sleep around nine hours a day and still wake up very tired; she felt exhausted after work despite not doing anything particularly physical in nature; she would then return home, sleep again for another nine hours, and once more awake not rested. This presentation is very vague; fatigue in a 40-year-old female can be due to any number of things, such as low electrolytes, pregnancy, thyroid problems, or even cancer. I needed to narrow this down, so I asked, "Do you take any medicines at home? And what for?" She replied, "I actually ran out of my medications for my thyroid and blood pressure a few months ago, and when I called my doctor's office back then they wouldn't refill it until I came by to see them; I didn't have the time back then and currently they are closed."

A wise doctor whom I trained with often said, "If you let the patient speak and listen, sooner or later they will tell you exactly what they have." Yet again, this proved to be the case. A confirmatory test revealed her thyroid levels were indeed low, and this was the most likely source of her symptoms. In this case, all that needed to be done was to restart her on her thyroid pills. Thyroid problems are quite common, affecting nearly 4 percent of the population over the age of 12 in the United States, and in Appalachia the rates are slightly higher at 6 percent. Left unchecked, low thyroid function could lead to confusion, swelling, and life-threatening heart problems requiring admission to the ICU. This is a clear example of a patient who suffered because of the pandemic: despite not having the virus, her condition resulted from policies made in response to the virus.

Another large number of patients were individuals who struggle with chronic pain—arthritis, a history of back injury or back surgery, or even individuals with substance abuse problems—and who are seeking relief from their pain. Unfortunately, the role of the emergency room is not to resupply patients with pain medication that they receive from their primary care providers; rather, its role is to screen individuals for medical problems that can be life-threatening if not treated in the hospital. Once the appropriate exams are performed, a decision can then be made as to where the patient should go next: Admit to the hospital? Or return home with instructions to see their doctor about their pain that is not life-threatening? For these patients, a tough conversation can ensue, as they will often leave without a refill of their pain medication and understandably believe that nobody did anything for them. Sometimes, the best help those who work in the ER can offer is to reassure the patient that "everything is OK; you don't need to be hospitalized; your medical condition is not life-threatening and your primary care doctor is the best person that can help you with this particular issue."

Another case is from a patient named Jordan (pseudonym) who came to the emergency room with complaints of leg swelling. The legs would "weep," a medical term for the bodily fluid that seeps out of a leg when there is too much swelling. This weeping will damage the skin and can cause it to slough off, exposing the nerves below it if not cared for properly; it may even lead to infections that become challenging to treat. Jordan had struggled with this issue for many years, with legs that required wrapping changes weekly to help the skin to heal. On the day she came to the ER, she was concerned that her legs needed a new bandage; she had no new injury, and upon examining her leg, we noted that she had the expected weeping appearance in her legs but without infection. She further explained to us that she had an appointment with her doctor for next week already scheduled, but she had not called her doctor to try and get an earlier appointment because the ER was "more convenient." That proved unfortunate because her leg swelling, while a serious problem in the long term, was not an acute life-threatening problem nor a medical condition that required hospitalization. Her needs would be better managed by her doctor, who knew her case, was an expert in leg wound care, and provides such care dozens of times a day, and not by an emergency room that is not designed to provide routine wound care.

I explained to Jordan that we would try our best to wrap the legs with new dressing but that a more ideal solution would be to call the doctor's office and request an earlier visit for this week. Her legs were cared for, and I made the call to her doctor's office, rescheduled the patient for two days in the future with her wound care specialist, and told her the appointment time. I was surprised to see that she was upset with me after arranging all of this for her; she said, "My legs are still leaking!" She left unsatisfied with her care that day. Such is life as a health-care provider; you never know who will walk through the door nor how they will leave. You can only do your best, and always try to do better the next time.

One weekend in the ER, a middle-aged man came to the emergency room complaining of "back pain." Back pain can be caused by a multitude of medical problems, anything from damage to the spinal cord to muscle cramps, injury to bones of the spine, pelvis, hip or leg, cancer, and even dehydration. Back pain can also be made worse by stress, depression, and anxiety as well as having poor coping mechanisms for the stresses of life. As explained above, EMTALA requires us to evaluate patients for serious conditions and make a determination if they need to be treated in the hospital or at home, so we did our due diligence to medically screen this man. A CT scan was performed showing no appendicitis, infection, or bone fracture. Lab work also came back normal for infection or dehydration. There was nothing visibly or palpably wrong with the patient's back, and he had no falls or recent injury that could explain his back pain. The only thing that seemed amiss was the visible discomfort he was having.

As we talked, I discovered that he had recently lost his job due to COVID-19 restrictions and shutdowns, and then he lost his home. He was living in his car and ran out of the pain medication that he would normally get from his doctor because he no longer could afford those medications. Unfortunately for him, there was nothing that the ER could do to help with his pain in the long term. We did help his pain with a combination of acetaminophen and NSAIDS, but in the long term he needed to be reestablished with his doctor, not only to manage his pain but to find help to deal with his life stresses that were likely making his pain worse, as well as to find a home to live in. There was no risk of loss of limb or life or underlying medical condition that needed immediate medical attention. His pain was very real, but the best care he could receive would be from his doctor. He, too, was unsatisfied with this assessment and, cursing all who could hear, left the emergency room to head back to his car to spend another painful and lonely night.

With time, it became clear that the peak for COVID in this region of Appalachia would not happen in March or in April of 2020. These months came and went without a major, sudden surge in cases, and the expected overwhelming number of patients with COVID-19 pneumonia didn't materialize. Our first COVID patient arrived in early April, and we never had more than five active COVID cases at the hospital until around October. Therefore, in June 2020, our hospital reopened the doors for families to visit their loved ones—with a limit of one visitor per patient in most circumstances; the dining area tables and chairs went back in place—with a limit of four individuals per table, six feet apart from each other. Elective surgeries resumed, floors dedicated to COVID were reverted to regular rooms, and our hospital and ER census slowly crept back up to just below normal levels. Some physicians here estimated that peak COVID cases in southwestern Virginia would occur around August 2020, and they were off only by a couple of months. As the end of the year holidays approached, that peak became a plateau. The winter of 2020 was our worst in terms of the number of COVID patients, and the things that were undone over summer—removing COVID-19 floors, allowing visitors in the hospital—were put in place once again. It was like a yo-yo of human emotions, trying to keep up with what the virus and hospital leadership were doing.

Even in early 2021, we were still seeing the effects of COVID-19 in the hospital: the cafeteria buffet was still missing in action; many nurses and providers furloughed in early 2020 found jobs elsewhere, leading to a worsening nursing shortage; many patients that I used to see in the clinic found a different primary care provider in the time I was out of the office, while others passed away from COVID-19. Visiting patients while wearing a mask has made it very difficult to communicate with those with hearing problems who rely on lip reading to understand. Despite all these changes, however, I have faith that our charming city of Abingdon, all of Appalachia, and the regions surrounding it will emerge postpandemic and return to normal—especially now that we have successfully vaccinated and boosted many in the community and continue to do so. We mourn those lost and others affected negatively by the pandemic and trust that better days are surely coming. Until then, all we can do is what we have been doing: our best, while trying daily to do better.

REFERENCE

1 Collins, M. *Carrying the Fire: An Astronaut's Journeys.* New York: Cooper Square Press; 2017.

# 7

## Shadrach, Sparrows, and Me

### TARA SMITH

*Editor's Note: Becoming a doctor is a powerful responsibility. What happens when the training module questions covering ethical and protective responsibilities during contagious outbreaks stop being philosophical? Dr. Smith speaks for many as she describes the soul reckoning that followed.*

"Beep . . . beep . . . beep . . ." The familiar sound of the cardiac alarm chimed from the collection of screens behind me. They monitor a handful of patients in our small intensive care unit (ICU) (just eight beds). I quickly turned my attention to them and away from my thoughts. I had been staring through a glass door into a COVID-19 patient's room. Phew! It was just a false alarm. A monitoring probe had fallen off the patient's chest, signaling the loud alert; no true emergency this time.

That COVID room I went back to after the false alarm was usually only covered by a cloth curtain. Because of COVID, it had been transformed into a negative pressure system that suctioned all air outside to avoid contaminating the hallway with this new disease. A large silver tube connected to the outdoors, tunneling air out. A man was lying in the hospital bed with tubes and lines tunneling around his body. His cheekbones were prominent, and he looked pale. I watched his chest rise and fall each time a breath was delivered from the machine he was connected to. He was frail. How could a microscopic virus that originated almost 8,000 miles away a few short months ago travel so far, so quickly? Especially to our sheltered Appalachia?

Despite the overblown drama of our profession as displayed on TV, I can attest that a typical workday can be very habitual, even in the high-stakes realm of the ICU. Of course, each shift has its own challenges and rewards, but as residents we are trained for every high and low. We're trained to handle whatever comes our way, be it boredom lulling one into a false sense of complacency, or a pandemic. Yes, that latter challenge was new, and a bit scary, but as doctors we signed up to expose ourselves to infectious disease in the hopes of saving others.

The day I looked through that glass felt to me just as dramatic as overblown scenes from hospital television. It was my first day back on the job since being personally quarantined. I was quarantined for the same reason this man was now here in my care: potential exposure in my case, actual exposure in his.

The word *quarantine* used to be a foreign concept bandied about in medical texts; now it rolls off everyone's tongues as part of their casual vocabulary. The last time the word *quarantine* seemed relevant came from a video game I used to play. What was it called? It involved avoiding cholera to advance in the game. Anyway . . .

A couple of months before I stood at that glass door, rooting for our patient to win his struggle to breathe, I stood at my apartment's back window, gazing out at the wintery landscape and making vacation plans. Travel for me can be an escape from reality. Growing up in a rural area of southeastern Kentucky, I was never exposed to many other places or cultures. Eventually, I realized that I could hop on a plane and be transported to an entirely new culture. From that moment on, every day of my 15 vacation days per year during medical training was spent in another land.

My mom is typically my partner in crime for these adventures. Throughout the past few years, we have slowly been chipping away at the map to see as many places as we can. We tasted the tobacco of Cuban cigars on the streets of Havana. We were led through the

Kuranda forest of Australia by a local to see wildlife grazing, not to mention a large python. We toured through the Colosseum of Rome, imagining what ancient times had been like.

Our tickets were booked in February 2020: from our little airport to a big one, across the ocean to Barcelona, and then on to Paris. Barcelona called to us with a beautiful beach and delicious tapas, while Paris is . . . well . . . Paris. It's my favorite city in the world. I could already taste the chocolate-covered croissants and hear the chatter of the most beautiful language.

My dreams of returning to Paris and exploring the streets of Barcelona came to a sudden stop when my mom called.

"Tara, I have the worst feeling about this. I've prayed about this trip, and somehow I feel so unsure about it. Isn't there a serious illness spreading in China? I heard it's in France now."

"Yes, Mom, that is true, but listen . . . I'm a doctor. This 'thing'"—my fingers made air quotes around the word, which she couldn't see—"has the same mortality rate as the flu. We wouldn't let that stop us, would we?"

Mom was unimpressed by my years of training and medical knowledge; she'd seen my bedroom as a child. "Tara, you're more willing to take risks than me. Let's just continue to pray about it."

That is a typical southern woman's response to any difficult situation, and I couldn't argue. So, we prayed. Each morning thereafter, I refreshed the news on my phone. Each day the numbers of those infected and dying doubled—and even tripled—overseas. The first American cases hit Seattle, just as we were making our decision on whether to fly off for sunnier climates.

Even with the spread of the virus into Europe and the United States, nobody in my area was concerned. Of course we felt safe in our little "Appalachian heaven," as my Texan friend calls it. Even when desperate things have happened in big cities of the world, we remained a peaceful place. As I asked for advice from my resident physician colleagues, consensus was mostly, without hesitation, "Go have fun on your trip." I know my colleagues are all very well informed, intelligent people, so I trust their responses.

Unfortunately, nobody could have foreseen what was to come. The most conservative response I received was to go alone and not take any children (which I do not have). I laughed, hoping my mom wouldn't translate that advice into a decision to go without me.

Mom and I agreed, after prayer and news watching, that a trip to Paris and Barcelona would be too risky. It might be safe to go on vacation, but not to such large metropolitan cities. Besides, Paris had survived so much over the centuries; it would be there when the pandemic had gone. We would go back then. We were dying for a trip away from the routine, but I really didn't want to risk one of us getting sick and turn "dying" into reality.

Still, that caution didn't mean we had to give up on our escape entirely.

"Let's go on vacation somewhere closer to the United States," I suggested to my mom.

There were at that time no restrictions on travel. Looking back, people may have a hard time remembering early March 2020, when that strange coronavirus was a "far-off" disease. It was largely confined to Asia overall and big cities elsewhere—or so we thought. Back then, the world minus those few places still felt like our oyster, Mom's and mine. Where could we go that would be close to the US with few to no COVID-19 cases?

"I've got it! The Caribbean! The sun will drown any microbes that we face and 100 percent of our worries."

My mom looked at me with a smirk. My attempts to impress her with medical insights rarely worked, but . . . "Tara, you know I've never said no to a beach!"

So we rebooked, this time for a cruise in the Caribbean with an all-you-can-eat buffet and a visit to beautiful islands, including Saint Lucia, Barbados, Saint Thomas, Tortola, and Antigua. I did the research. There were no cases of COVID-19 on any of these islands. What could possibly go wrong?

Many things could go wrong, it turned out—horribly wrong. Hindsight is always 20/20, but something about that white sand can be quite blinding.

Saint Lucia was beautiful. Barbados was beautiful as well, but by the second day of our trip, news began to filter in that the world back home was falling apart. On the ocean, there's very little connection to the internet, so we relied on bits and pieces of news we saw on the one channel available in our cabin and from information exchanged during spotty phone calls with family.

My sister called around day two and told us that there was a national recommendation that no one should be traveling by cruise boat. Talk about timing. That same day, the bar stopped self-service, which was very unusual for a cruise. While on a boat ride in Saint Lucia, we were told by the tourism company how happy they were to have us, as so many other cruise boats had not arrived. My mom gave me a look. I swallowed hard, and smiled back. *Medical professional here, nothing to see. . . .*

Clues followed on clues, but it was too late for Mom and me to admit the mistake we had made—okay, *I* had made. We were in the wrong place at the wrong time, and all we could do was pray—which we did.

Meanwhile, family members back home reported that there was no toilet paper or hand sanitizer in grocery stores. How could this be? Before leaving on the trip, I went into the grocery store as normal and picked up one of many bottles of hand sanitizer on the shelf. Now the stuff was a rare and precious commodity?

The morning we were meant to visit Puerto Rico, where we would depart the boat to fly home, our situation took a turn for the worse. Around 6 a.m., the captain's voice came over the intercom. In a surprisingly panicked tone, he told us that we were not allowed to disembark the boat, as there was concern we might infect the citizens of Puerto Rico. He said we would be quarantined for 3 days, maybe more, and we were now heading back to Orlando to end our cruise. He also assured us that nobody on our boat of 4,000 people was sick.

My stomach turned. I feared the worst: that our boat would be quarantined for 14 days. We'd seen on our cabin's news channel the infamous reports of the *Diamond Princess* quarantined at sea. We had no window in our cabin, which was only a bit larger than your average parking space. Would we lose our health and our minds in that tiny dark room? If one person developed COVID-19, I now understood, then it would only be a matter of time until my mother and I would as well. How could I have exposed her like that? I couldn't have imagined her getting sick in the middle of the ocean. She had me, a doctor, close by, but to what advantage? Would I know how to help her but not have the proper tools and medications available? What would that feel like?

Imaginations can be both blessing and curse.

We prayed. With almost 24-hour access to an all-you-can-eat buffet that never shut down despite contagion terrors, our stomachs proved too nervous to eat those extra two days on the boat as we cruised to Orlando. The growing feeling that we would be stuck on that boat against our will even after arriving in Florida was slowly drowning us in dread. We spent the next two days doing what we could to keep our mind off things. We exercised in the gym. We watched the free movies that played in the common areas. We woke up very early the day we were docking in Orlando in an attempt to be at the front of the exit line.

Our captain spoke over the intercom again. Mom and I braced ourselves for impact as his words would reveal our fate. "We have been accepted by the port authorities. No temperature checks. We will call you all out by floor to exit."

It was a miracle. I don't know that I've ever heard sweeter words. Forget romantic talk from a potential suitor; I was just a girl who wanted to go home. I wanted to go back to work and care for my patients. I wanted to give my dad and sister the biggest hugs. I wanted to hold my dogs, Teddy Boo Bear and Chloe Chanel. I wanted to live in a normal world again.

The world was no longer normal. Little did I know, I wouldn't be seeing my family or my patients for weeks. I wouldn't be able to give my dad or sister a hug. Shortly after stepping off the boat, I received word from my manager at the hospital where I am a resident: go home and quarantine for 14 days. During my absence, being on a cruise boat had gone from "no big deal" to a level 3 COVID-19 threat.

Okay, so it could be worse. This is not the end of the world, I told myself. We could have been stuck on that boat in our sunless parking-lot room for two weeks. Someone on the boat could have been sick; we could have gotten sick. I had my dogs and my familiar apartment and my computer for continuing my education, plus communication with friends.

But things in this new world were so different than I had left them. My sister dropped off toilet paper for me (without ever seeing me), as every store was empty. Who knows where she was able to find it? I didn't ask questions. I recalled several cruise passengers slipping it into their bags from the boat.

Day by day, I served my time in my small apartment. Friends dropped off food now and again at my doorstep. I worked from home mostly by studying, making PowerPoint presentations, and doing practice board exam questions. I ironically made a very detailed PowerPoint on the disease process of COVID-19 to present to my fellow residents. My program director and manager worked very quickly to make sure I had learning material to last for two weeks.

In fact, I enjoyed the time I had to rest from the most stressful vacation of my life. I spent each day by the laptop with a dog on each side of me. So little was known about COVID-19 at the time that I was even hesitant to be around my dogs. I had heard some reports of dogs catching the disease but not actually having symptoms. I had to take my chances on that one. I was sure my furry companions believed I had been fired from work, and they liked the idea of that—more time for them.

When my 14 days were over, I was permitted back into the hospital. In residency, we never stay in one area of the hospital for too long. We live our lives in four-week intervals called rotations. Each month we head to a different department and try to soak up knowledge and experience there, whether that be the ICU, a regular hospital floor, the emergency room, an outpatient clinic, or a specialty service like gastroenterology, cardiology, or neurology.

Of course, upon my return from quarantine, I got sent straight into the heat of the battle—the ICU. This battle unfortunately was no longer just for our patients and their families; as health-care workers, we now had to manage our personal fears of contracting this sickness.

So little was known about the virus then. With the circulating stories of COVID-19 claiming the lives of healthy young people on the news, I wondered each day, was I going to be next? Would I be a victim rather than a health-care hero? My coworkers and I regularly discussed the pandemic around us. What were the odds that one of us would become infected?

Our residency cohort could be described as very tight-knit, one of those rare groups that turns out to be more sympathetic than competitive. We only have about five people per graduating class, with only three cohorts at a time, as residency is three years. Some months we may spend 288 hours together. Those 288 hours are broken up into 12-hour workdays, six days a week. After that much time together, we're no longer friends. We're family. We work as a team in the hospital, and there's nothing we wouldn't do for one another. We have laughed until we cried together to blow off steam in the middle of a rough day. We've listened to one another when times get difficult. Nobody wanted to see a fellow resident get sick.

Sometimes the anxiety felt overwhelming. This mental battle was something not to be taken lightly. COVID-19 was no longer a disease affecting those 8,000 miles away. COVID-19 had come to us. It came lightly at first, in small clusters that we considered "the big spike" each time they happened. We had no idea, that spring and summer, how much worse it could get, which was probably a good thing.

One night before starting back to work, I opened my Bible to whatever page it flipped to, as I have many other times. That night it opened to the story about Shadrach, Meshach, and Abednego. I read that these men were walking through the fire, yet somehow, miraculously, they weren't burned. Okay, so it was another Bible story I've known since I was a child. But this time, the story really stuck with me. I continued to think about it as I worked, studied, cleaned, played with the dogs, and mentally prepared to go back to work again. I knew God was telling me, *This is you. You will be in the middle of the fire, cases of COVID-19 all around, and I will sustain you, as this is what you are meant to be doing.*

Our ICU is set up sort of like a wheel. The computers that residents, doctors, and nurses alike use are in the center of a large room, flanked by smaller rooms all around the edges. The computer I sit at throughout the day is about 15 feet from the closest room.

Back to my first shift postquarantine, I was looking at the patient through the glass door. This glass door was connected to the closest patient room to my workstation. This patient—let's call him Vince—happened to be a 72-year-old man who had just returned from a missionary trip to the Caribbean. He had been helping to develop a school in a low-income area. I was unable to touch his hand and assure him that everything would be okay, as we sometimes do. Our hospital administration had decided that in order to lessen the spread of the disease, residents were not to enter the room of a positive COVID-19 patient. We were still following their progress and putting in orders for their care, but we could not physically walk into the room.

As I looked at him, I was honestly embarrassed to think how this man had spent his time in the Caribbean compared to how I had spent mine. He was an inspiration. He had worked most of his life in coal mines, where he had developed coal-worker's pneumoconiosis, known medically as silicosis. That is an honest living here in the mountains. Sure, it's risky. It's not uncommon for a man to die inside a mine or to slowly develop lung disease from everyday inhalation of coal dust; either way, the mine kills.

My dad was a coal mine inspector. I remember as a young child seeing stickers he would bring home to place on the fridge about prevention of "black lung." Because I'm a physician, I understood the pathophysiology and prevalence of this disease; and because of all that those little fridge stickers represented, I understood the life of this hardworking, caring man in the hospital bed. I said a prayer for Vince, standing there feeling guilt, fear, peace, hope, and lastly gratitude that I might be able to help him in some way.

Vince wasn't the only victim in our hospital. A few short days later, I heard the chatter of the nurses in a hushed tone: "Here comes another." Moments later, in a louder tone I heard, "He's crashing!"

Sitting at my computer screen, I immediately checked for newly arrived patients to our ICU team to research the emergency en route to us. I scrolled down the list; there he was, 90 years old and admitted from a nursing home.

I breathed out an instinctive prayer: God have mercy on us. If he was from one of the nursing homes in our little town, it was only a matter of time before the entire population in that facility became infected; that much we knew already about how this virus worked. We saw it happen in Seattle as residents in a nursing home became sick one by one, then in New York City. Nursing homes were like cruise ships with frail passengers, plus harder to seal and faster in spread.

All right then, it was time to fix this guy. As the nurses transported our 90-year-old patient to ICU, I scanned his records: past medical history, past surgeries, family and social history, and the symptoms that brought him to the emergency room. Mentally, I had been keeping track of symptoms, whether it was runny nose, sore throat, or fever. We had heard reports on television about anosmia, or lack of the sense of smell. There were no reports of that around here. I wanted to keep a record of symptoms positive patients had so that no cases slipped by me. It used to be so easy as a physician to throw a diagnosis of common cold onto a patient, but not anymore. How would we learn to differentiate these symptoms from the common cold before it's too late? Before the infection spreads from 1 person to an average of 2.5 others, and from those 2.5 to 5 more, and from there . . . you get the picture. We sure did—the television news kept blaring it.

This nursing home patient (let's call him Gus) was peculiar in that his symptoms were not related to his upper respiratory tract. Gus came in with diarrhea and vomiting. Another point of anxiety for providers—COVID-19 may present with a wide variety of symptoms, making it even harder to diagnose. I noted the symptoms Gus exhibited for the running list in my head. It wasn't until after being admitted that his oxygen levels began to drop. That's what I saw next in his chart: oxygen saturation in the 80s, even though he was on the highest amount of oxygen we could give without putting him on life support. (It should have been well above 90.)

Another problem arose. We wanted to get Gus onto the life support he needed with as minimal exposure to the health-care workers around him as possible. We call this "intubation," and you could say it is a very intimate process. Typically, one person, usually a doctor, will stand above the patient, hold the patient's mouth wide open with what we call a "blade," and slowly direct a tube into the patient's lungs through the wind pipe. This tube is connected to a machine that delivers oxygen to the patient. It is almost impossible to accomplish this without breathing the air the patient is expelling.

I watched as a respiratory therapist brought out a large, clear plastic box. I'm not sure where it came from or what its originally intended purpose was. It looked like the type of box a baby lies in at the neonatal intensive care unit. It had perfectly round holes just the size for a hand to fit through on each side. I watched the ICU-trained physician put on his gear to enter Gus's room. He deliberately placed each item on in the order that we've all been instructed: shoe covers, gown, mask, eye cover, gloves. He placed his hands in the clear box over the patient and guided the tube into his lungs. A small crowd of nurses, residents, and respiratory therapists gathered outside to watch. This was something new in our pandemic world, and we all wanted to learn. If it were to get bad enough, I thought, any of us might have to do that procedure.

A very somber mood settled over the ICU for the next few days. Yes, Gus had access to the life support he needed, but nobody wanted to see him that sick at his age. Each day he seemed to get worse. We knew by then that the elderly and those with preexisting medical conditions were most at risk for a poor outcome with COVID-19. Gus was living proof.

After lengthy discussions between the care team and the man's family, a decision was made. He had suffered long enough while breathing by a machine, and it was time to let him rest. Shortly after being taken off life support, Gus passed away.

I continued to press on. It's all any of us could do. Vince was still on life support in another room. He was receiving doses of azithromycin and hydroxychloroquine. Hydroxychloroquine is a medication that received a lot of hype in the mainstream public for a short time, especially while I was working in the ICU. As a doctor, I associate it mainly with treatment for autoimmune diseases like lupus, or it is sometimes used to treat or prevent malaria. We have a few patients in the clinic who take this medication regularly, but it is a very small number. I don't have a lot of experience prescribing this drug, it being mostly prescribed by a rheumatologist or an infectious disease specialist.

I heard different opinions about hydroxychloroquine before it became such a hot topic on the news. One of my attending physicians really likes to use it for rheumatologic disorders as it has significantly fewer side effects than other medications that treat the same condition. An ophthalmologist I know hates the retinal disease he has seen it cause when used long term. Nevertheless, we were giving this medication a try for our lingering COVID-19 patient Vince. In his critical condition, it was one of our last hopes to help him. Hopefully, giving it for such a short amount of time would decrease his chance of side effects if he were able to pull through.

I checked the news app on my phone and saw reports of President Trump saying that hydroxychloroquine and azithromycin seemed to be a promising treatment for COVID-19. I wondered about that to myself. Yes, I am a clinical resident and not in research medicine, but how could an antibacterial medication like azithromycin have much effect against a virus? Still, azithromycin has been shown to have anti-inflammatory properties as well, so hey, it was possible. In a desperate situation such as this, with his wife's permission, we had to try it. If we don't try everything we can, a patient may not make it. Vince was in that position.

In residency I'm taught to practice only evidence-based medicine—that is, medicine proven by clinical trials to benefit a patient in some way. We normally have tons of resources available to us on any given medical topic, but we did not for COVID-19. This novel virus is called COVID-19 for a reason; it first appeared in humans in 2019. There were few to no trials of medication used against this virus in any of the online databases I usually turn to. How do we practice evidence-based medicine without any evidence? In this new world, we are the scientists. We are the investigators. And I was a second-year resident.

It was May 2020, and to be quite honest, that is when our patient load normally declines a bit. As the weather warms, illnesses begin to fade away. Because of the pandemic, we had even fewer patients; people were afraid to come to the hospital. Day in and day out, we kept an eye on our sole patient, Vince, to make sure he was optimized. We adjusted his medications and ventilator settings as needed.

By that time, most of my personal anxiety had faded. Wearing a mask for 12 hours at a time was no longer a foreign concept. Before this pandemic, N95 masks, the kind that will block particles as tiny as the flu, were in abundance at every patient door. The pandemic caused a nationwide shortage, and soon each room had only a box of thin surgical masks. N95s were given to those in direct patient contact.

Back home before bed on a May night, I opened my Bible randomly again, and it was once more the story of Shadrach, Meshach, and Abednego. How kind God was to show me those verses again; I remembered the assurances of not being burned while passing through fire and slept peacefully.

The next day, sitting at my usual computer desk, I heard the same muttering from the nurses that I heard the last time we had a new positive COVID-19 patient. But this time, I heard "in his 30s" and "works in health care." Immediately, I worried that it was one of my fellow residents; why else would someone in their 30s be coming to the ICU? Was anyone really safe? I drew a deep breath; God had said I would be. That had to count now.

I never knew the details of this patient's case, which was great news. As an ICU team we residents didn't see everyone in the ICU, only those who were either extremely ill or needed life support. Since we were not called to see him, he never required life support. I also learned that he was not one of my fellow residents. I never really knew if this patient had a lung disease that may have predisposed him to being more vulnerable. I wish I had known more about this case, but I am glad that our help wasn't needed.

He left on the same day news came that one of us was infected. When I say "one of us," I mean a staff member that I had likely interacted with—one who was fearless on the front lines caring for patients and who used the same work space all of us in ICU used.

Thankfully, my fellow staffer had only mild symptoms and was not admitted like the 30-something who spent days in ICU. The staff member was sent home to get well and quarantine. Who would be next? Would it be my coresident, working beside me in the ICU? Had we been careful enough? I began what would become a ritual that evening on arriving home after work: I dropped my scrubs and shoes at the door, wearing a second pair of clothing underneath; went straight to the shower and scrubbed. This entire process took 30 minutes, including sanitizing my phone, cleaning the doorknobs (dropped from the routine that fall), and placing my dirty scrubs in a bag all tied up and waiting to be washed on the weekend.

My mom, dad, and sister were all a few hours away in Kentucky and temporarily uninvited to my possibly infected apartment. Would all this be enough? I remembered the Bible story I had only recently read, and again I was comforted.

Every day in the ICU we tried to wean the patients from life support. First, we would stop the sedating medications. After the patient would start to wake up a bit, we had to know they weren't in any respiratory distress. We checked that the respiratory and heart rates were normal—check, check, and check for Vince. After all this, we asked them to cough. This let us know their ability to protect their airway from their own secretions. We also asked them to follow a simple command such as a "thumbs up."

"Sir . . . please give us a thumbs up, sir," the nurse yelled into Vince's ear. His chart indicated some difficulty hearing before he came to us. She raised her voice a bit more than she typically did, practically screaming to elicit a response. With a very feeble hand, Vince slowly but surely raised his right thumb into the air. I watched in amazement as the patient with the coal-damaged lungs breathed on his own and smiled.

I couldn't help but feel an overwhelming surge of hope and happiness. We fixed this guy, I thought to myself with satisfaction. He was taken off life support later that day, and then transferred to a regular unit in the hospital. I didn't have any more hand in Vince's care after that.

It was a couple weeks later when I heard a song playing over the intercom system throughout the hospital. It sounded like an old folk song with possibly . . . wait a second . . . that definitely *was* a banjo. I had been working at the hospital for two years, and I had never heard a sound like that before over the intercom.

A few employees rushed to the window to look outside. I followed in curiosity. Down below, walking out the front door of the hospital to greet his waiting family and head home, was Vince. A videographer filmed the moment as staff members cheered him on from windows and doorways. The song playing over the intercom was selected especially for his departure, Vince's favorite hymn, "His Eye Is on the Sparrow." Staff members up and down the corridor began singing along.

> I sing because I'm happy
> I sing because I'm free
> His eye is on the sparrow
> And I know He watches me.[1]

Do I have to tell you that we were all bawling like babies?

My experience going from a normal hospital to a pandemic hospital was almost literally overnight because of the ill-fated cruise Mom and I took. For me, there was no gradual progression to a new way of doing things. I came back from my vacation to a new world that we're all still learning to navigate. By the time of my fourth week in the ICU, we no longer had any positive cases in the unit, and the total number of cases in southwestern Virginia was dropping.

We knew that this was round one with COVID-19 for all of us. We very obviously were not suffering to the extent of those in our larger US cities, such as New York, Chicago, and Los Angeles, but any life lost here in our small community is one too many. COVID-19 came at us for real in late fall of 2020. Vaccines started rolling not long after. Delta reared its ugly variant head a few months later, the first of many to follow throughout the waves of infections in 2021 and 2022.

Come what may, we treat our patients with the best medicine possible, and as always with supportive care. In COVID cases, supportive care included ventilators, infection control plans, and caring people who play special hymns when our patients depart.

Whatever is to come as we slowly emerge from this global health threat, may I always remember that His eye is on the sparrow, and there is no fiery furnace where He cannot be.

REFERENCE

1 Martin, C.D., Gabriel, C.H. His eye is on the sparrow. In: *Revival Hymns.* Chicago: Bible Institute; 1905.

# 8

## I Am Responsible for the People Who Are Responsible

TAMMY BANNISTER

*Editor's Note: Rounding out graduate medical education perspectives, a residency director in northern Appalachia details concerns regarding surge timelines, concerns for learners, and hospital economics. Rural Appalachia's experiences were markedly similar within itself, unremarkable to high population areas where infection waves rose in rapid succession. Did rural Appalachia have less resources to fight with, fewer infections to fight, different dangers than urban zones, or something else? What patterns do you see emerge from Appalachian pandemic accounts?*

A flood warning, a tornado watch, a chemical spill alarm: these are the closest comparisons I can think of that nearly equate to the COVID storm in which we found ourselves in March 2020.

The first warnings seemed far in the distance and not necessarily applicable to us here in Appalachia—similar to MERS, SARS, Zika—all scary, all real, but very little impact here locally. During the early days of 2020, I was ramping up information to teach residents about the presentation of illness to add to their differentials (as in, how to differentiate symptoms shared by multiple seasonal diseases) and how to initiate care until confirmation of whether they were dealing with COVID-19, not flu or sinus infections. It all seemed academic.

Then the rumblings of thunder sounded closer: illnesses in California, Washington, and New York—still far off and a bit difficult to be relatable here, but discussions turned toward protecting the public and the health-care team. Would we have enough personal protective equipment (PPE)? How would we limit travel and still allow residents to get elective training? I started teaching how to don and doff PPE. Our meetings and lectures were almost all about COVID-19. Our group didactics (i.e., classroom education rather than hands-on lab or clinical sessions) changed to cover immediate issues such as Centers for Disease Control requirements for quarantines and travel bans, who was at risk, and how to protect yourself and your family. That might have been the first time I saw it begin to dawn on the residents, the strange new world that was headed their way.

The thunder grew louder and the rain started and so did my anticipatory anxiety: How would I protect the residents if they are seeing patients? How would I instill the importance of PPE and its preservation yet not cause a culture of fear? How would I maintain their well-being—physical, mental, and emotional? Oh yes, and beyond keeping them well, how would I continue their education during a pandemic?

That sounds ironic, but how could I make sure they saw enough patients during this time to graduate? How would I ensure they had broad training sufficient for them to pass board exams? Their electives were all closed; how would I make sure they had some educational experience during the months that health-care volume was so low in all other areas, yet climbing, climbing, climbing in just one?

Patients started coming into the clinics with COVID-like illnesses. OK, now what were we going to do? The hospital was set up to test; we needed the same precautions and more. Residents had slowly become aware that beyond coronavirus causing disruption in their training to some extent, it was also a real risk to their health and the health of their families. We began to rethink all our normal processes in clinics and the hospital: residents would change clothes in the office in order to decontaminate before going home; we would separate hospital rotations from outpatient care to minimize cross-contamination; and we needed to decide who would be involved in the care of those patients who were sick with COVID-19.

Each resident's situation was unique; some were pregnant or had pregnant wives, several cared for elderly family members, a few had travel plans for away rotations, a couple were out of the country when things got serious, and it is fair to say that most were anxious. As the person tasked with keeping them safe, I tried not to broadcast how much I worried about them.

It became clear we could not continue our usual workflows. Residents were limited to non-COVID patient encounters in the hospital, but who knew what kind of symptoms might come into the office during walk-in hours? In order to limit resident and patient exposure risk, we developed a tent process for screening/testing patients and implemented these stations at every entrance to the hospital and clinic. The tent process also limited overuse of PPE and allowed residents to participate in the decisions and care of potential COVID patients; their patients were still their patients, but if they came with COVID symptoms, they did not get an opportunity to infect others.

Everything going on in the clinics and hospital seemed to revolve around COVID. I started worrying that we would be missing other common disease diagnoses in our high-risk Appalachian population. Everything that causes a cough and shortness of breath is not coronavirus; remember black lung, COPD (cardio-pulmonary disease), and other prevalent illnesses in West Virginia? Residents recognized that many of their vulnerable patients might be at increased risk for complications from their chronic illnesses if they were not able to come into the office for in-person visits. We started a process to call and check in on them, making sure their medical needs as well as other needs were being met. Food insecurity is real in our population, and the shutdown of foodbanks and other supply lines exacerbated it.

It took us all a while to relax our grip on "all things COVID," but as we worked the tent and ramped up telehealth visits, residents and faculty alike returned to the broad-based training we all knew and added COVID-19 symptoms to our long differential list.

Our residents were very adaptable to the changes in the office setting and workflows; as soon as we were able to provide telehealth visits, each resident went through a brief training and checked off a competency list. That done, they were off caring for people in our community again with the direction and backup of faculty—who were learning at the same time how to use new technology; how to teach our elderly patients to use their smartphones, if they had one; how to document and bill in this truncated staffing situation where telehealth was the new normal. It seemed nearly impossible that a bunch of doctors who hate paperwork could accept, let alone learn, this new system when we started, but within a week we were excelling at it. Managing chronic medical problems, adjusting medications, diagnosing new problems, and treating depression, anxiety, rashes, and more online wasn't in our playbook when we became medical professionals, but adaptation is the first key to survival. In this case, that survival encompassed our patients.

During all this change, I started meeting with my resident advisees weekly, checking in on their anxiety levels, home management, and workflow. How was their job hunt going for when they graduated? How were they managing childcare? When did they think their spouse would be called back to work? Did they have adequate space at home to decontaminate and quarantine if needed? Were they feeling overwhelmed? Concerned about graduating on time? For those who lived away from our area, how were they handling being separated from their family? Was there anything they needed?

They seemed to be doing better than me. Their grace under pressure, ability to hold together multiple life stressors, and capacity to focus on the job at hand were nothing short of astounding. "Don't worry," I was told over and over by these young, strong, capable people. So, I switched to worrying that I might be projecting my own concerns and anxieties onto them.

Thankfully, we had limited cases of COVID in our part of West Virginia, until Thanksgiving ended. It gave us time to prepare. Our residents who were slated to graduate have done so and have launched into brave new careers in a strange new world. Those then in their final of the three required years were still learning, still teaching me courage, and still providing excellent care to their diverse patient population through telehealth and in-person visits. They were vaccinated. Someday this will all be over, and all our residents will be the stronger for it.

# 9

## Isolation, Denial, and
## Appalachia's Greatest Public Threat

### NIKKI KING

*Editor's Note: Health-care specialists in the field of substance use disorder redoubled efforts to keep up with those trying to leave this disorder behind. In a branch of medicine whose mantra is "The opposite of addiction is connection," what were the ramifications of enforced isolation for the greater public good, and how did care providers feel about that?*

When the first reported positive COVID cases began to emerge in the United States, they were on the West Coast, far away from folks cradled safely in the Appalachian Mountains. So as news of the novel coronavirus broke, to many of us here in Appalachia, it was just one bad thing that happened far away to people they would never meet—a view largely encouraged by local and national political leaders.

By summer's end in 2020, the full-blown pandemic had joined a cacophony of apocalyptic-esque happenings across the nation. Black versus blue lives, election violence, and murder hornets dominated the airways, carrying tales of terrible events that again barely affected the people of the mountains—although some were coming closer. Many residents of the coalfields live in communities too rural to garner protest marchers, with more still being able to count on one hand their number of encounters with law enforcement. So it was only natural that many assumed COVID would pass them by as well.

It didn't.

COVID had ripped a path of destruction from sea to shining sea, leaving spiraling death rates, widespread food insecurity and outright hunger, and a general collapse of social safety net programs. Food banks closed alongside small businesses, a cruel irony. Those who suffered the greatest impact of the epidemic were marginalized groups with preexisting economic insecurities and chronic health conditions. That was particularly true of people with substance use disorder.

When news of the statewide lockdown reached Autumn Campbell, she was working as a peer support specialist for a recovery center in Kentucky. Autumn's position relied on her reaching out to individuals who were struggling with substance use disorders and connecting them to recovery communities where they could find support, social engagement, and treatment opportunities.

However, as the mandatory lockdown brought daily life in rural Kentucky to a grinding halt, Autumn saw a significant shift for the worst in most clients. Many church services were canceled—an essential lifeline to those whose substance use disorder had left them socially and emotionally isolated.

"People who are struggling with addiction really need routine, they need a support community, and they need accountability," Autumn said, "and when COVID hit, all of those things went away." Autumn knew this story all too well, being in recovery herself for two years prior.

"I was raised in a good family. A God-fearing, Christian family with both parents. We didn't live in poverty or anything like that. There wasn't any kind of abuse. I had a lot of friends in school, I loved sports, I had a great childhood," Autumn recalled. "But the anxiety was always there—the depression. When I got to college, I guess you could say I was kind of sheltered. I was so desperate to fit in. I got enmeshed in the partying lifestyle, and before you know it I couldn't stop."

Autumn remembered her turning point as standing in front of a judge who told her that he believed in her, that she had value, and that he knew she could change for the better. While she was involved in the criminal justice system, she connected with peer support specialists who helped her find a renewed sense of community and purpose.

"Without meetings, going to church, meeting with probation, having jobs, many people who are in addiction struggle to find purpose. When COVID hit, many of the people in recovery lost their routine, and we all know that drugs numb those feelings." According to Autumn, many people who were, for the first time, making headway in their recovery journey faced significant setbacks. Those who were active in addiction fell further into the hole as their last remaining connections withered away under social isolation.

In the summer of 2015, British journalist Johann Hari postulated, via a scorching monologue delivered as a TED Talk, that "everything we know about addiction is wrong." He described the research that has since become known as "Rat Park," a series of studies on drug addiction done at Simon Fraser University, in British Columbia, during the late 1970s. The general concept is that rats involved in a study on illicit drugs were significantly more likely to show symptoms of addiction when isolated and understimulated than those who had adequate social interaction and more activities to participate in. Hari connected the study's theme with our modern understanding about substance abuse disorders, their cause, and anticipated treatment. There are several nuances to the Rat Park theory, the likes of which have drawn both acclaim and ire alike from those who confront the substance abuse epidemic. While the overall implications of this study may be widely debated, critics and fans agree on one thing: no one is made worse off by feeling socially connected and integrated into their community. From troubled youths to lonely seniors, meaningful social interaction and engagement is the recipe for improved mental health.

Welcome 2020: How do you continue to socially engage populations who are at increased risk of harm during a pandemic?

For many, the answer to this question falls on the backs of some of the pandemic's most critical but often overlooked essential workers: social workers, community health workers, and volunteers. In an environment where 30 out of 50 states had reported sharp increases in opioid overdoses in 2020, the effect of social isolation on those struggling with substance abuse disorders was clear.[1] Aside from further ostracizing individuals who already struggled with isolation based on a poor reputation in the court of public opinion, the inability of peer support groups such as Alcoholics Anonymous or Narcotics Anonymous to safely meet eliminated the first line of defense that saw so many individuals safely to recovery.

"We're definitely seeing an increase [in substance abuse activity]," said Candance Gentry, a social worker on the front lines in southeastern Kentucky. She also noted that, while the activity had been slowly tapering down since the beginning of the COVID-19 crisis, the hardest part of recovery in the region had always been the persistent lack of resources to address patients' needs. COVID bringing an increase in the number of people struggling with mental health concerns exacerbated that problem. When the region couldn't get patients the care they needed precoronavirus, it was a given they would be struggling even harder in the midst of the pandemic.

"We only have one homeless shelter in our region, and it's a whole county away. They serve such a large area, and with social distancing, they've had to cut down their volume. It's like that everywhere—inpatient facilities, shelters, drug and alcohol treatment programs, they're all cutting capacity to keep people safe." Gentry explained further that the precautions made sense (especially with so many individuals having underlying health concerns), yet they highlighted a problem that already existed.

Michele McCord, who works at the West Virginia domestic violence shelter Hope Inc., echoed many of these sentiments. Michele noted the difficulties in rotating staff and client services in order to follow protocols and keep everyone safe; however, she, too, noticed the stark increase in referrals during the crisis. "The increase in volume of people needing help increased drastically in the beginning," she said, "but the really unusual part was the intensity of the patients. All of the people we serve need our help, but these clients were incredibly challenging—a lot of needs."

Together, McCord and Gentry conveyed a similar tale of a region already buckling under the weight of a strained social safety net suddenly being overwhelmed with need. Increases in domestic violence, homelessness, substance abuse, and food insecurity left many frontline care workers paralyzed to meet the needs of the patients in front of them. "We got everybody taken care of in the end," Gentry said of their efforts to provide safe housing and basic necessities, "but sometimes I didn't know how we were going to do it. It was so hard to get everyone where they needed to be."

The pandemic was a new challenge for the Appalachian region; the high levels of strain on the social safety net due to the prevalence of mental health and substance abuse challenges were not. A survey conducted in 2008 of 410 Appalachian counties in 13 states showed a level of severe psychological distress higher than the national average and higher than average incidence of conditions like major depressive disorder. Hospital admission rates of opiates and other synthetic substances of abuse were similarly shown to be higher in Appalachian regions, with a particularly high intensity in the coal-mining Appalachian regions. Surprisingly, Appalachian regions were found to have competitive access to treatment for individuals seeking substance abuse recovery services, with intensive outpatient programs being some of the more popular options.

Intensive outpatient treatment programs (IOT or IOP) have long been tried and true in the mental health and substance abuse arenas. This comes as little surprise given the cost associated with inpatient treatment facilities. Unlike traditional outpatient programs, many intensive outpatient programs focus on treating not only substance abuse disorders but also underlying psychiatric disorders, while assisting the patient in addressing social challenges. These programs are typically between 9 and 12 hours of therapeutic intervention per week and rely heavily on group psychotherapy to provide social support to those struggling with addiction. In particular, group psychotherapy has been noted by the federal Substance Abuse and Mental Health Services Administration to have several advantages over other modalities. These advantages include positive peer support, real life examples of people in recovery, positive social interaction, family-type interactions that are often more supportive than the patient's home environment, and peer confrontation and discipline to build insight.

One of the most powerful benefits of a group is the "uh-huh, yeah, sure, whatever" moment. Inevitably, in most patients' journeys to recovery, they hit a stage of prolonged sobriety. Often this period (especially if it is the patient's first significant experience with sobriety) is accompanied with a false sense of confidence. "I haven't used it in over a year. Besides, alcohol isn't my drug of choice. It should be fine if I go to a bar with my friends," says the patient. In their mind, their sobriety is iron forged. They have collected key chains, they have participated in recovery walks, they have helped shepherd others into recovery. However, when the patient is engaged in group therapy, they are invariably met with the "uh-huh, sure, yeah, whatever" moment from the group. If they're very lucky, this is followed up by a barrage of stories of those in recovery who, when met with similar situations, unfortunately discovered that sobriety is more of a journey than a destination when their high-risk behavior precipitated a relapse. If the patient is very, very lucky, something someone says will sink in. The alternative is that a clinician, likely without their own recovery history, advises a patient against an ill-advised situation at the risk of seeming judgmental or unsupportive of the patient. There is great power in storytelling circles where someone will say, "We've all been there, we've all made that same mistake."

That power disappeared during COVID.

There are multiple types of recovery groups for individuals with substance abuse disorder. The highest level of care is a partial hospitalization program (PHP), which is led by a qualified therapist and psychiatrist eight hours a day, five days a week. IOPs are slightly below PHPs in intensity of care, with nine to twelve hours a week of therapist-guided clinical services. Outpatient therapy, consisting of either a single one-to-three-hour group per week, one individual therapy session, or some combination, is the lowest intensity of therapeutic services. Recovery groups, such as Narcotics Anonymous or Alcoholics Anonymous, constitute a separate group that often runs parallel to clinical services. Despite the level of service the individual qualifies for, there is one common thread: all rely on the power of leveraging social integration strategies to help build healthy, prosocial thinking in individuals with substance abuse disorder. Unfortunately, the same strategies that made these groups such a potent form of treatment also made them a hot spot for spreading the novel coronavirus.

The most logical and immediate response of treatment providers in the face of crisis was to move all possible services online to protect both patients and providers alike. However, this presents some challenges that are universal, and a few that are rural specific. One of the difficulties with online treatment options across the board is providing crisis services. For example, a patient who is trying to engage in telephonic or telehealth services may be homeless and thus cannot locate a private space. In an individual setting, this presents a threat to the patient's privacy and potentially even safety. In a group, this is even more challenging because it presents the same problems, but it is multiplied by everyone in the group.

Additional challenges have included individuals who do not have access to wireless internet at home. These individuals may try to engage in services in public areas with Wi-Fi access, such as a McDonald's or Starbucks. Again, this compromises patient privacy and security, not to mention it costs money out of pocket to buy a burger or a coffee. The challenge of inadequate internet access is even more poignant in rural communities, where access to broadband and cellular data is significantly limited. According to a report released by the Federal Communications Commission, 39 percent of people living in rural areas lack access to broadband internet as opposed to just 4 percent in urban areas.

In addition to challenges with internet access, rural communities often lack sufficient transportation systems. Most communities do not have access to bus or taxi services, even if insurance products, such as Medicaid, provide reimbursement for the trips. Having transportation for patients not only includes the expense and upkeep of owning a car; it also means the patient will need to have access to a valid driver's license, a privilege that is often revoked as a result of substance abuse–related convictions. Another transportation challenge that is specific to the Appalachian region is its dispersed nature of housing. It is not uncommon for individuals to commute to their remote town center from an even more remote location, known as "hollers." These hollers, which typically provide more affordable housing options, can be 30 minutes or more away from the local town, which is where the treatment providers are typically located. Particularly in the case of intensive programs such as IOPs or PHPs, this amounts to a significant amount of travel time and resources for these individuals. Much of this resource cost for the patient can be mitigated by wireless treatment options—if they are available. While certainly not perfect, lowering the barriers to treatment oftentimes means that individuals can focus more on engagement and treatment goals.

Of course, while providing treatment in patients' homes reduces barriers to care by removing the need for extensive travel resources, it assumes the patient has an adequate housing situation to be conducive to treatment. This means not only stable and consistent access to internet services and a home that is free from domestic violence, but also a home that has enough resources to be warm in winter and food security year-round. When people talk about rural America, often one's mind conjures idyllic images of family farms and cellars brimming with food. However, the reality is often far from that image. Individuals who experience food insecurity are shown to have poorer health outcomes and health indicators across the board.

While battling food insecurity, like many safety net resources, was seldom enough to meet the need in rural communities prior to COVID-19, it came to a crisis point early on in the outbreak. "We have a lot of folks who come into the hospitals and places here and they don't have enough to eat. It's sad. We try to do what we can for them, but it is so hard right now," Gentry said. Social distancing requirements affected food supply systems nationwide, forcing closure of churches and other small volunteer organizations that hosted community food banks or dispersed other resources, leaving many who relied on those supplies without another option. Additionally, transportation, where offered, now had reduced capacity to bring individuals to places where they could acquire food. Virus concerns and staffing challenges shuttered many small, family-owned grocery and convenience stores, even without a direct order.

In this quiet and insidious way, the "election virus" (as many people in rural Kentucky had taken to calling it) began to rack up damage long before it ever crept its way into the mountain hollers. However, by fall, it had arrived in rural communities in earnest. The lifting of the lockdown did little to augment the failing safety net. Recovery groups began meeting in person again, only to have large swaths of participants go out sick for weeks at a time, or voluntarily quarantine (one hopes) due to becoming symptomatic with no access to testing. Churches and treatment centers resumed services, but beneath the veneer of normalcy, smoke began to rise.

By November, the hospital system serving Appalachian Tennessee and Virginia began reporting large spikes in positive cases. One in six of those cases would end up fatal. Across the state line in Kentucky, roughly half of the rural eastern counties had already shuttered their community hospitals before the pandemic was even a rumor at a faraway airport (see chapter 1). Those now facing the wrath of the virus they had staunchly believed would not come for them—some because they thought the mountains were too isolated, others because they preferred to believe it didn't exist—were an hour or longer away from the nearest emergency room.

And yet, perhaps emboldened by President Trump's seemingly miraculous recovery, many remained ambivalent, even as the numbers rose into the double digits.

"When it finally does come to this community, I'm afraid it's going to go through here like a wildfire," Gentry predicted in June

2020, months before local hospital representatives dominated local news sources, pleading with the community to practice social isolation to stop the spread. She was right.

What does that "We got nothing to worry about" attitude toward the pandemic have to do with substance use disorder treatment? Denial is a big part of addiction. One of the first things you must confront is believing that you are an addict. Perhaps denial proved to be equally devastating amid the pandemic. Isolated, alone, and denying that there was a problem, people in rural communities have died alone, in hospitals in cities hours from their home, swearing they didn't have the virus—or a substance use disorder. Rat Park has come to the mountains.

### REFERENCE

1 Coady, J.A. Preventing overdose and death. Substance Abuse and Mental Health Services Administration, August 31, 2021. https://www.samhsa.gov/blog/preventing-overdose-death.

# 10

## The Mask Makers

*How Women in Appalachia Were Empowered through*
*Sewing during the COVID-19 Response*

MELANIE B. RICHARDS AND MILDRED F. PERREAULT

*Editor's Note: Previous articles focused on professional health-*
*care workers; now read how community members fought the*
*pandemic as individuals. Women in Appalachia have tradi-*
*tionally been in charge of family health; this reached a new*
*level of expression during the pandemic as they took up needle*
*and thread. Two researchers stitch together the voices of 15*
*Appalachian women to tell this story.*

Mask makers are amateurs and artists. They are primarily women: mothers, daughters, grandmothers, community members, and workers. They are creative and resourceful. They are bound by where they live but also redefining community beyond place. For all these women, making masks seemed like a natural response to the COVID-19 pandemic. As the pandemic went from a possible crisis to a reality that required many people to stay at home and socially distance, this step helped them feed their desire to do good for others while employing self-efficacy and making a tangible impact. When COVID-19 required a massive adjustment in the way they lived their daily lives, people in communities across Appalachia began to do what Appalachians do best: band together (from a safe social distance), use the resources they could access, and take action where they could.

BACKGROUND

On Friday, March 13, 2020, the US government recommended people shelter in place in response to the COVID-19, or coronavirus, pandemic. Throughout Appalachia, health organizations began to ramp up efforts for response, repurposing funding and supplies. While the impact of COVID-19 was yet unknown, people had begun to return to the region from travel and tell tales of the virus. For example, an Elizabethton, Tennessee, physician and his wife, both in their 70s, were quarantined in Japan for many weeks after the wife contracted COVID-19 while aboard the *Diamond Princess* cruise liner.[1] In total, 700 cases were confirmed aboard the ship they were on, with 3,711 passengers and crew members on board.

Talk about the virus, which causes serious respiratory disease, had been in the international conversation since late 2019, when cases appeared in Wuhan, China. Though research now supports that the virus was already in the United States in late December 2019, the nation did not have a strong reaction to the disease until several months into 2020.[2] By early March, concerns had surfaced, with cases quickly saturating larger cities like Los Angeles, Seattle, Washington, DC, and New York. State shelter-in-place orders were primarily the result of the inability of hospitals to treat their regular patients and the additional number who were expected to be admitted as a result of COVID-19 complications. People began to get scared and bought up supplies like toilet paper, masks, and hand sanitizer in bulk, as well as groceries for the next few months, to avoid going to stores. Hospital administrators and workers also began to worry about limited access to masks and other personal protective equipment. Local news organizations attempted to provide targeted and accurate information to their communities despite misinformation.[3]

For months, the US Centers for Disease Control and Prevention (CDC) had said people needed to wear face masks only if they were ill or were treating people who were ill. This was because most scientific studies found that basic medical masks do little to protect wearers, and instead primarily prevent sick people from spewing infectious droplets from their noses and mouths.[4] The World Health Organization (WHO) generally agreed with the CDC recommendations during this time period. However, during the first week of April, the WHO updated their recommendation to include that people other than health-care providers wear masks if the person was sick or interacting with those who were sick.[5] The CDC in America changed its stance on mask wearing around the same time to align with the global WHO recommendation.

During a health information conference in early April, President Donald Trump announced that people should use a cloth face covering when they visited crowded places as a precaution, although he would not personally be following the recommendation.[4] This recommendation aligned with the WHO guidelines as they evolved further in early June, with the organization then recommending that the general public use cloth masks in confined or crowded public areas and those over 60 or with preexisting health conditions wear medical masks when physical distancing proved impossible.[4]

In the Appalachian region, many were already concerned about the pandemic, especially with the associated predictions of overrunning hospitals with cases of severe coronavirus patients.[6] Americans in rural areas tend to have a higher rate of smoking, high blood pressure, obesity, and similar high-risk diseases, which make people more vulnerable to severe cases of COVID-19.[7] Health risks, access to health care, and a shortage of health-care workers were common rural challenges even before the pandemic; thus there was a concern among many that the disease impact could be particularly harsh across the region. At the same time, they began to worry about the economic impact, as shutdowns crossed the country.

In response to their health concerns and looking for some form of protection, many people attempted to follow the evolving guidelines and find masks—only to quickly realize that both online and physical retailers were completely sold out. In response,

Appalachians evoked their recognized technique of making do, meaning making the most out of what they can access when ideal resources are not available.[8]

In the case of masks, this making was quite literal. Mask makers in Appalachia became part of a national mask-making trend, driven primarily by women. How they went about sourcing materials, distributing finished masks, and sharing support for their communities through mask making is a case study in resilience and community spirit.

### SELF-SUFFICIENT AND INTERDEPENDENT

Appalachia is a mountainous region that spans 13 states in rural, suburban, and urban communities.[9] The traits of self-sufficiency and dependence were ingrained in the culture of the Scotch-Irish mountaineers who settled in the Appalachian region in the late 1700s, and this juxtaposition continues to be central to the Appalachian community.[10] Historically, Appalachian people have worked to make do or do without by expanding resources when they are strapped and reusing old items to make broken things work again—what Porter and Richards have termed radical resourcefulness.[8,11]

Studies have also examined how Appalachians learn and pass down culturally specific skills through the generations while also using these skills to care for their neighbors.[12] Health and economic advocacy and action have appeared in Appalachia and other rural communities in times of community and regional crises.[13,14] This balance between self-sufficiency and helping one's neighbor is frequently associated with Appalachian culture and identity.

### HEALTH DISPARITIES IN APPALACHIA

In Appalachia, access to health care is of great concern. People living in rural areas may be more than 30 miles from a health-care provider and even farther from a hospital.[15] Lack of health insurance or being underinsured are deep concerns for people living in Appalachia.[16] In the past 10 years, several studies have identified higher rates of cancer, heart disease, premature mortality rates, and other health conditions, which put this population at greater health risk.[7] The Appalachian Healthcare Cost, Coverage and Access Index showed that counties in the Appalachian region have more health-care cost, coverage, and access disparities than many other states.[17] While the percentage of uninsured persons under age 65 in the region (15.8 percent) is slightly lower than the national average (16.8 percent), there is high enrollment in Medicare and Social Security disability coverage.[17]

Appalachians are resourceful people accustomed to looking for solutions, many of whom recognized the challenges of COVID-19 to current health disparities, as they did other health threats. So finding a way to respond in a crisis proved vital for a population with a slightly higher risk of contracting the disease than many American communities.

MASKS, EMPOWERMENT, AND STIGMA

When people face a crisis, they often seek to do something tangible to help themselves or others. Similar actions of self-efficacy and empowerment have been seen in wartime, with the planting of victory gardens and women taking up jobs that were held by men in World War I and World War II. This was recognizable when women reused materials during the Great Depression to assist in hard economic times.[18] Women have also been known to spearhead movements concerning health issues by holding drives and public events,[19] as in the issue of breast cancer.[20] Empowerment-related actions appear both during immediate crisis response and as a form of long-term crisis resilience.

Self-efficacy in crisis has been linked to the central goal of mitigating harm and sharing information, a function served increasingly by social media when on its best behavior.[21] The five-stage Crisis and Emergency Risk Communication Model assumes crisis events develop along a somewhat predictable pattern. In this model, the second stage involves the initial crisis event, which is hallmarked by uncertainty reduction, self-efficacy, and reassurance.[22] In stage three, the maintenance or mitigation stage, the goal is to further reduce uncertainty. During this stage, self-efficacy and reassurance also build. Also, communication during this time involves connecting people and resources. The goal is to empower the public toward actions that will help them manage the crisis individually and communally.[22]

Coping theories from psychology and sociology also speak to this desire to have an action that helps those facing a crisis to take control. Taking concrete actions has been found to help people gain a tangible way to cope, as this allows an individual to see beyond the challenges to reassert control over circumstances.[23,24] Masks are something tangible that could reduce risk in a health crisis, and making masks is a tangible action to enact risk reduction and communicate concern for others at the same time.

Despite these benefits, research on the public perception of mask wearing in the United States during the H1N1 epidemic in April 2009 found that most people did not feel a strong compulsion to wear a mask given the risk, with only 4 percent of people agreeing that wearing a mask was a preventative measure.[25] Even with the practice being somewhat normalized internationally in areas where large groups frequently congregated in public, prior to COVID-19 many people assumed mask wearing was to protect the people wearing them, not those without masks.[26] Studies have found that grassroots health campaigns can work to curb stigma and empower people to change their behavior in relationship to health risks and crises.[27]

SOCIAL MEDIA AND CRISIS COMMUNICATION

Social media allows for people to communicate about risks and share their actions and adaptations, which can be especially beneficial during times of crisis. Many health and crisis engagement campaigns use social media to share information, gain engagement and followers, and elicit crisis response.[28–31] Social media campaigns that are successful help define community by allowing participants to express part of themselves to others.[32] This is because social media can be personal and rewarding in that it provides instantaneous connection and response. Social media messages communicate with certain groups about topics of interest. The action of sharing information in a crisis not only helps people to communicate with their communities but also advocates for a specific stance. Though a person's primary goal may be personal benefit, in this research we examine usage for community good.

WHAT WE SET OUT TO LEARN

To better understand how mask making became part of the response to the COVID-19 crisis in Appalachia, we wanted to hear how those who made masks interpreted and reacted to the situation and what they took from the experience. Here is the guiding statement we settled on for this informational storytelling journey: *learn from mask makers' own accounts of their lived experiences in order to better understand perceptions of what went right and wrong regarding homemade mask making during this time period.*

As supplemental questions to that guiding statement, we asked the following:

- How did mask makers view public conversation about homemade mask making and usage during the COVID-19 epidemic?

- What was their perception of crisis communication regarding homemade mask making?

We were fortunate to find 15 women willing to hold in-depth interviews via Zoom web conferencing. All interviews took place in late April through early May of 2020. Recruitment took several forms, including public social media posts on both Facebook and LinkedIn and via email referrals. The mask makers we spoke with live in northeastern Tennessee, southwestern Virginia, northern Georgia, western North Carolina, and southeastern Ohio, with points between. Some referred to themselves as transplants, while others were lifelong Appalachian residents. Given our location in northeastern Tennessee, we don't give significance to these locations; they radiate out from our university.

One Latina and one Black woman participated, the rest identifying as White. The women ranged in age from early 20s to early

70s, and their work situations varied. Though most older makers were retired from their full-time jobs, many still worked or volunteered part-time. Younger and middle-aged makers worked either full-time or part-time. Several had experienced a disruption in work due to the COVID-19 pandemic, while others had been deemed essential and continued to work, either from home or at their regular location. Consistent narrative themes emerged when we analyzed their interview transcripts using elements of grounded theory methods, including inductive reasoning, field notes, and open and axial coding.[33,34] Each theme is listed under its own heading here.

### MASK MAKING AS WOMEN'S WORK?

All the mask makers interviewed identified as female. We did not set out to present the experience of males who sew in Appalachia, but anecdotal experience leads us to believe that female dominance in mask making could also be considered as a finding. Sewing is still stereotyped as women's work by many, despite the fact that the

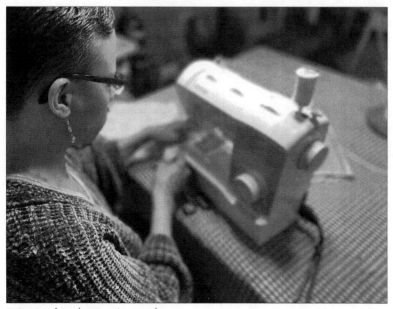

FIG. 10.1. A maker creates masks.

historical occupation of tailor has been male dominated.[35,36] Women interviewed could not recall any men in their respective social circles who were making masks, yet they did call out men serving in a variety of helping roles: cutting fabric, pinning, providing supplies, and taking on additional household duties, such as a greater share of childcare, so that they could use that time to make masks. Some mentioned recognizing the stereotype of sewing as women's work, but they did not feel that taking on this work diminished their power. Rather, it was another way to harness it.

> I think part of it is generational sexism. I remember in the seventh grade, when we did our electives, that they automatically signed up girls for home economics and boys for shop. So, we were on the tail end of that. We still had very sexist division of labor. (Lisa)

> I like getting my hands dirty. I like doing work. I like people to know that women can do work and we are here to do it. But at the same time, I also like doing the more stereotypically femme things like sewing. I want to be a strong woman, but I also want to still be creative. Just because I'm a femme woman doesn't mean I'm not a badass. (Leah)

Every mask maker interviewed had some level of experience with sewing prior to making masks for the pandemic, but these levels differed. Some considered sewing a routine part of their lives; others hadn't touched a sewing machine in years. Several described professional sewing work, such as an alterations service or quilting business. Some described themselves as artists, others as crafters, others as hobbyists, and still others didn't describe themselves with a title or role name at all; sewing is something they *do* versus something identifying who they *are*.

## APPALACHIAN, NOT ISOLATED

Another prevalent theme emerged: these women felt that Appalachian doesn't necessarily mean isolated. The stereotypical image of a hillbilly living in a wooded, rural holler, with little connection to the outside world, has evolved alongside global technological advancements, particularly with mobile data connectivity and expanding broadband, cable, and fiber internet services becoming the norm. More than 70 percent of Appalachian households had a broadband internet subscription according to the 2013–17 American Community Survey Findings.[37] All 15 of the women we spoke with could access online resources, with a few using this global connectivity for employment purposes. Many knew what was going on in other countries early in the COVID-19 news cycle and started planning for what might be needed when the pandemic's effects eventually rippled into their own communities. Several also had family or friends in other areas that were affected earlier or family that served in government or medical roles whom they trusted for up-to-date information.

> I teach English to Chinese kids, and the virus starting in China really affected that part of my life first, because the kids—they have been on lockdown, like legit boarded-up apartment doors, government hardcore lockdown, for a long time. And because of that, they were taking more online English classes. . . . So I was a little more acutely aware of it. (Tricia)

> I have family who live in New York City, so I was getting some information. They were concerned. My nephew and his family were able to leave the city and go to an area that was a little safer. (Gwen)

> Initially, I was hearing about it because friends of ours had parents on the ship outside of Japan, the *Diamond Princess*. So we had a pretty clear idea really early on that it was something to take seriously. That it was heading our way. (Lisa)

> My son was out in Seattle. Early on, the piano teacher came to the house to give my six-year-old grandson a piano lesson. And she said to my daughter-in-law, I just don't feel well and my husband's even sicker than I am.

> And my daughter-in-law said, I think you should call your
> doctor, and lo and behold, they both had it and they ex-
> posed my daughter-in-law and my grandson. (Betty Ann)

> It was frustrating to me that they were suggesting the
> average citizen doesn't need a mask or the average per-
> son shouldn't be wearing them in public. That was really
> frustrating because what I was hearing from the parents
> [I work with] in China was "Don't leave home without a
> mask; you should absolutely have a mask." . . . Also, my
> brother works for the Department of Defense. He doesn't
> know a lot ahead of time, but he knows more than the
> average person does before we do. . . . And my sister, being
> a nurse practitioner, takes care of elderly people. (Mandy)

Many Appalachian mask makers saw themselves as globally
connected. In this vein, they viewed their ability to make masks as
something that could help fill a need in the region, as well as beyond, by shipping them to family, friends, and others in more distant locations.

### INITIAL PERCEPTIONS: MASKS FOR SELF-PROTECTION

Respondents had varying perceptions of masks based on their own
prior exposure and usage. Prior to the COVID-19 pandemic, most
had understood that masks were something used for self-protection
from potentially harmful biological or environmental elements.
Some had previously worn masks themselves for protection. Mask
wearers were generally perceived to either be ill themselves, have
a compromised immune system, or to reside in areas where pollution was particularly bad. Several mentioned that they associated
mask usage more with other countries than with the United States
before the pandemic, either because of perceived cultural norms or
air quality reasons in specific geographies.

> I probably [thought] they had an autoimmune
> disorder—that they themselves are sick or could easily be
> sickened. (Leah)

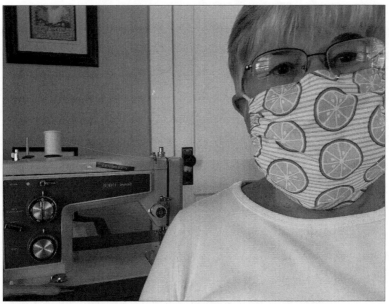

FIG. 10.2. A maker wears one of her creations.

You saw someone occasionally wearing a mask. I usually
just assumed that they were someone with an immunocompromised system. Going through chemotherapy or
maybe they had asthma. (Melanie)

I was thinking they're hypochondriacs and they're trying
to protect themselves. They're just scared of germs. Now I
think a lot differently. (Edie)

We visited Vietnam after we got married, probably 15 years
ago, and in Vietnam and other Asian countries people wear a
mask all the time, because there's dust everywhere and they're
mostly riding bicycles and scooters and motorcycles. (Tricia)

I had always thought of mask wearing on a regular basis
as something that people do in places where there's lots
of air pollution. Say, some of my friends who come from
Asian countries where mask wearing is a regular thing in
big cities. . . . Whenever I would see somebody wearing a

mask I would think, well, there must be a reason that they are wearing that. That means that they either have a health problem or something is going on where they can't tolerate either the air or pathogens the way that most other folks can. (Cara)

It's a little bit comforting for somebody who has asthma and autoimmune issues that it's no longer taboo to wear a face mask when you leave the house. (Abbie)

Though initial perceptions of mask wearing varied, all understood that masks were for protection. Masks could also be employed at an individual level of action, providing a greater sense of control and self-efficacy.

### INFORMATION INCONSISTENCY

As it became increasingly certain that COVID-19 would directly affect the United States, people began to look for protective measures to ensure the safety of family and friends, as well as their own. However, the firehose dissemination of information coming from all angles was inconsistent at best and blatantly conflicting at worst. Individuals became overloaded with mixed messages around mask efficacy, types of masks, and how to use them. The mask makers looked to recognized experts such as the CDC and WHO for information, but they also supplemented that knowledge by consulting experts within their own personal networks and searching online for valid information regarding mask efficacy (including filtering materials).

We were hearing that the N95 were what you needed, but they weren't available. (Nancy)

It just seemed like there was so much information, so much differing opinion. (Abbie)

The CDC was not recommending masks—"You don't need to have a mask, you are okay, please stop buying N95 masks, please stop buying these medical-grade masks." But then it switched, and they updated it to say, "Hey, no, you should actually wear masks. The cloth masks don't protect you, but they will protect everyone else. Your mask protects other people and other people's masks protect you." The president is telling us something. The CDC is telling us something. This guy sitting in his house is telling us something. This doctor is telling us something else. You're getting 50 different messages. It's hard to sift through, and it takes a lot of time to sift through it. (Shea)

It was kind of a train wreck because they recommended no masks for us to begin with on the basis of health professionals needing them, which was true, but that doesn't satisfy a person's need to protect themselves. And so, there was some distrust there for sure. I think that has affected the number of people that are wearing them now. I still see a lot of people not wearing them. (Melanie)

We should have started from the angle of "Reach out to your local crafters, or if you're a crafter yourself, here's what you can do to protect yourself and your family." If we started from that . . . we would have all been protected much sooner and more effectively and then there wouldn't be this stigma of there's no reason I should wear a mask. Everybody says they're not effective anyway. (Mandy)

My brother-in-law is an infectious diseases doctor, so I was fortunate to have advice from him about what level of personal protection was appropriate for the work that I do and the interactions that I have. (Lisa)

Facebook is a great source of information and misinformation. (Bonnie)

In looking at all the YouTube tutorials and things, you go down that rabbit hole and there's like a bajillion videos. You read all the articles and you know how inundated you get with information, whether it's good information or not. (Cara)

While the information around masks has changed since the CDC first initiated shelter-in-place recommendations, most people see limiting the virus's spread even a small amount to be of benefit. However, the information inconsistency and evolution over time caused many in the general population to question cloth mask efficacy and therefore refuse adoption.

### SELF-TAUGHT

While the mixed messaging delayed some and motivated others, once mask makers committed to their construction they quickly realized that they were entering uncharted territory; there wasn't just one way to make an effective mask. Makers again employed self-reliance and researched which approach they would use for mask construction. Several consulted the CDC. Some used patterns received by email from a local quilt shop or handed down from another maker. Others followed the pattern made more widely available by specific national chain craft stores. Still others researched and watched countless videos on YouTube. As they made masks, many continued to source information, including from other mask makers, on how to make their masks even better over time.

> [My friend] would post a video, and then she would tag me on it. But then sometimes that video was not enough for me, so I would go to YouTube. I would search how to make masks with ties. And then when I needed to do the filter pocket, I searched for YouTube videos that could help me make the pocket insert for the filters. (Sonny)

> I started looking at the CDC website, spent a lot of time on Pinterest, seeing what the recommendations were, what it was actually supposed to look like, how it's supposed to fit. (Shea)

> A quilt shop that I follow on Facebook posted, "We think we're going to need to be making face masks because there's a shortage of the N95 kind, so we think we need to be making face masks. Here is an array of different

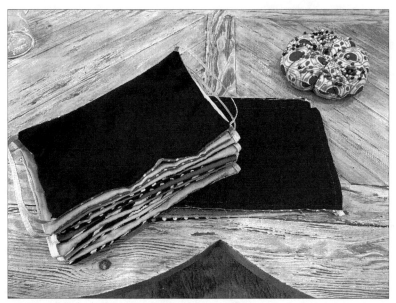

FIG. 10.3. Masks in progress.

patterns that we think might be useful." [The hospital system] has also asked for masks. They sent out a really detailed pattern for two different types of masks and those are really the patterns that I've been using. (Abbie)

Sew the Curve Flat [provides] several mask patterns. (Nancy)

A friend happened to mention something about seeing it on YouTube. I also looked at the [hospital system] website and looked at the CDC website. The CDC website says two layers of fabric, and [the system] wants two layers plus interfacing. (Gwen)

It's a bit early in the game to really have peer-reviewed research. So some of it is just common sense and trusting your source. (Lisa)

Even when they encountered inconsistencies in the available in-formation, the mask makers said they remained committed to their work. They received patterns, made their own, and passed patterns along to friends and family members as well.

### RADICAL RESOURCEFULNESS

Once they began the process of making masks, the women realized that many supplies were going to be difficult to source. Most had a significant amount of fabric on hand from prior quilting or sewing work (known as a stash), but elastic was also required for many of the available patterns, and most stores were sold out. In addition, an interfacing material dense enough to be an effective moisture barrier was a desirable component most planned to incorporate. Again, this was in short supply. Wire to build the nosepieces of the masks and even thread also began to sell out in many stores.

At this point, many mask makers began to display radical resourcefulness.[37] Some ripped seams from old pajamas and used a utility knife to salvage the elastic; others did extensive research and learned that landscaping fabric is a great and abundant source of dense polypropylene for interfacing and that chicken wire can be used for nose pieces; still others found a new purpose for flimsy hair ties. Many learned that their families, friends, and community members were more than happy to pitch in the resources they had readily on hand to help in the effort: a few pieces of fabric here, half a spool of elastic there, a few extra sewing needles, even a sewing machine shipped from a family member across the country.

> We pride ourselves on our fabric hoards. We have these collections of pretty things that we've held on to forever. But yeah, it's all gone. . . . Interestingly, the nonwoven polypropylene [for interfacing] . . . I found a very good source for that that is very abundant, especially this time of year. It's landscaping material. . . . It's the same density, if not a little bit better, than a surgical mask. I learned that you can shred T-shirts and it makes the softest earpieces. . . . It has good stretch, but it also has good recovery, so it won't get saggy over time as soon as you wash it. It just snaps back to that original shape. (Mandy)

One thing that we did since we couldn't find elastic, someone started doing them with the women's hair ties. Someone tried to use the regular black ones, and you know how stiff they are when they're brand-new. And then someone found a package at the Dollar Tree that were more flimsy, and flimsy in this situation was better. Because they could extend more and they weren't hurting people's ears. (Sonny)

Neighbors have given me some elastic, and I took apart all my old pajamas in the rag drawer, any clothes you don't wear that have little pieces of elastic. I just use my little X-ACTO knife and stripped off the sewing and it was clean and usable and worked. (Bonnie)

I have discovered that I can cut up my old stockings and tights. You take strips of that and if you give them a stretch, they roll up into a little roll and they make perfect little ear loops. (Melanie)

One little old lady, a wonderful friend of mine, she found me over 10 yards of elastic in her sewing basket, and other people the same way. (Betty Ann)

This cord, it's really thin clothesline. The fabric stores were out of everything. So this is clothesline that I bought at the hardware store. (Gwen)

This focus on using what is available is consistent with other traits found in Appalachia. Using what one must to make the greatest impact, sustainability of and repurposing of materials, and even making them fashionable are consistent with Appalachian culture and identity. This also conveys a sense of both authenticity and humanity and amateur aesthetic in the final product.[37]

PROMOTION AND REACTIONS

Mask makers got the word out about their efforts via social media (primarily Facebook) and through word-of-mouth efforts. Most

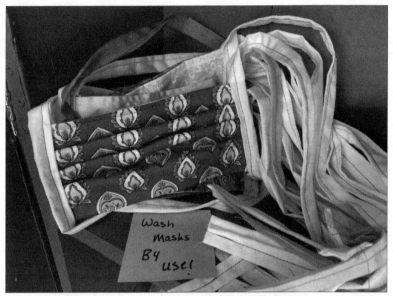

FIG. 10.4. Masks donated via a free community pantry box.

initially started making masks and distributing them to family members, close friends, neighbors, and fellow church members. From there, several looked for organizations in the community (e.g., hospitals, nursing homes, doctors' offices, ministries, nonprofit organizations) where they might donate masks to make a positive impact. Some made them for their coworkers and wore them to work. Some sold them to companies so that they might provide them to their employees. Some made less than twenty, while others made more than a thousand. Masks were distributed through contactless pickup on a porch or in a newspaper box, mailed to family and friends in other regions, and dropped off at homes and businesses.

> They've all gone to friends and family because I have been busier than normal. I just don't feel comfortable committing myself to more masks than that. Life is stressful enough right now. (Abbie)

> Because I quilt and I have all this fabric that's available, I decided I can make these masks, send them to my family

in Puerto Rico (who were already pinging me through Facebook that they can't find them). So initially it was just for our immediate family. (Sonny)

I just put out the word through my church that I was going to do this and if anybody had supplies they wanted to donate. A lot of people have things just [sitting around] and this was a way for them to participate. Then one of the members of our church runs the River Ministry downtown for women, and she let me know that they were going to need a lot of masks once that ministry reopens, because people come in there to do laundry and congregate and they're a very vulnerable population. So that's where I think most of my masks are going to go. (Gwen)

My mother-in-law, she visits the Cancer Center for her husband, and they were in need of masks. So I told her that I would make them to donate, and then I just ended up making some to sell as well. . . . I posted it publicly on Facebook and then I also used my alterations page to share it to those people as well. (Amber)

For individual health-care workers, I've given them theirs for free. And then [for a] corporation—they offered, "Let us buy these from you." I feel like it's a company's responsibility to provide them for their employees, so I don't feel guilty about that. (Mandy)

While most reactions to mask making were positive, some received criticism when wearing their masks in public or through social media posts featuring their masks. In response, mask makers would either ignore or attempt to correct perceived misinformation.

[After making a mask for a friend's child,] one of her friends [on Facebook] commented, "This is worthless, you might as well not even wear it. . . . It's like 10 percent safe." And so I was able to copy and paste the article from the

CDC that said it was closer to 50 percent and that something is better than nothing. (Sonny)

I had one friend who said, "I'm not going to wear this, because it doesn't protect me," and then another person said that they weren't afraid of the virus. (Shea)

I've gotten a lot of rolled eyes and things of that nature. I've had people who have purposely approached me and tried to stand in my space in a kind of aggressive stance; that happened a couple of times in parking lots of the grocery store. They sometimes have something to say like, "Your mask won't protect you." In that instance, I just said, "This isn't for my protection. This is for your protection." (Melanie)

We stopped to pick up an order at [the store], and a man was there just skipping through the store with no mask on, taunting people and saying, "I'm so scared. I'm gonna get the COVID." Some people I know have said, "I will never wear a mask. You can't make me wear a mask. #freedom." Someone else said, "You think that mask is going to protect you?" And I said, "No, I think it's going to protect you." That was a good way to shut that down. (Lisa)

The very act of wearing a mask can create a reaction. Even though there were some negative responses, more typically respondents found it caused people to become more interested in the mask or in wearing one themselves. For most respondents, making masks and wearing masks went hand in hand.

SOMETHING IS BETTER THAN NOTHING?

Despite many personally using and advocating for masks, at the time of the interviews several respondents mentioned that they still didn't know how effective the cloth masks really were. Some had made peace with the idea that something is better than nothing, while others felt uneasy about this. There were also open questions for some that had donated masks to organizations regarding their utilization. They worried that the masks might be put aside some-where in a box or a closet and never actually used.

> We don't know to what degree it actually does protect people. We do know that it does reduce the amount of transmission right now at this point. Even with the press conference, the president said, "Hey, you should probably wear a mask." The CDC recommended that. So, it's kind of interesting how that's changed a little bit. (Edie)

> There's so many different sources of legitimate informa-tion that I really don't think there's any right and wrong, other than not wearing one at all if you're close to people. Confusion can make people feel like, I'm doing something right. Or I'm doing something wrong. And I don't think that's helpful at this point. (Gwen)

> [Where I had been donating,] I was told that the person who was collecting them was going to decide how to use them. And I thought, well, I'll wait until you decide what you're going to do with them. I haven't stopped officially, but haven't given them any for a while. . . . I wonder about whether or not they're useful, or just some fad or craze. (Betty Ann)

Despite the inability to know precisely how effective masks were at that time, most respondents felt empowered by the mere action of making something and contributing to the possible prevention of the disease.

### TO SELL OR NOT TO SELL?

Respondents had mixed perceptions on selling the masks they made. Many had no intention of selling, for various personal rea-sons, while others saw mask sales as an opportunity to replace lost income due to negative employment impacts. Some didn't place a price tag on the masks, but decided to take monetary donations, and used that money to cover materials. For those who decided to accept monetary donations, many were surprised to find that the donations they received were very generous. Of note, all who sold masks mentioned trying to price them as low as possible and also donated a portion of the masks they made.

> I made some for myself and made some for my family [and other people who've asked]. I've not had anybody pay for any of them. (Cara)

> For me, it's a very personal thing not to accept any money for it because I know people don't have it. All the cloth except for the lining was [Teresa's, my mother-in-law]. It's kind of a way to keep the kindness and the love that Teresa had, keep it passed on after she's passed away. (Shea)

> They're not perfect and I'm using a lot of found materials around the house. I just don't feel like I ought to charge for this sort of thing. (Melanie)

> [I was donating them all and] they were saying, "I would gladly give you $10 for each mask." I said, "You know what, that's fine." I'll go ahead and do that and that way, in the future, when things get to some kind of normal, I can hopefully recoup my fabric back. (Sonny)

> People are just so generous and so happy. Sometimes when you don't set a price, people give you more than they would have if they were paying for them. I'm going to keep putting it all back into supplies until there's no need to do anymore. (Tricia)

> A big thing is not having to worry about my own security financially at this time because things are changing so rapidly still in China [where my work is based] that I don't know whether my schedule is going to be filled or not. I don't know what that's going to look like. (Mandy)

> I'm a potter who works commercially making whole-sale pottery for different businesses, and our business

completely dried up almost overnight. It was really a matter of see a need, fill a need. I saw this need and I had the skills and the materials to do it. Initially, it was friends and family who needed masks, and then it just expanded by word of mouth. For me this will put food on the table for my kids right now, so this is where I need to focus my energies. Financially, it's been a huge help, even though we've been doing pay what you will. (Lisa)

This isn't my job. It's really a hobby, almost self-care for me. It's soothing, calms me. If I were to take money for them, it could start down a slippery slope of this becoming a job and not being enjoyable for me. (Abbie)

While the long-term making of masks at or below cost might not have been sustainable for some, others said they only made them to give them away. If mask wearing were to become more common and the market grew more saturated with mask products, several said they would plan to specialize in certain types of masks or no longer provide them at cost or for free.

## MASKS AS FASHION

From March through May 2020, masks evolved from functional protective gear to a still functional but also fashionable outfit accessory. Well-known apparel companies positioned at various points on the price spectrum also went into the business of making and selling masks. Mask makers mentioned receiving requests from people wanting it to match their outfits, display favorite sports team colors, a logo, a mascot, or even to match wedding colors for a bridal party. One of the respondents had a clothing business and used leftover fabric to make masks that matched the vintage shirts she was already turning into crop tops.

Some mask makers were not interested in taking on the extra work required to customize masks (especially if they were donating them). Still, the general perception was that this was a positive trend that would can encourage greater adoption of masks in the future.

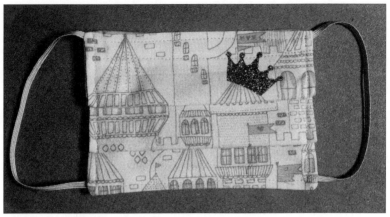

FIG. 10.5. A child's custom mask.

A few respondents also specifically called out the impact of unique and fun patterns on children's mask usage going forward.

> Everybody is using a mask for a fashion statement. And I was thinking, I have my little puppy dogs [fabric]. If a doctor or a health-care worker shows up and they have little puppies all over their face, it will make it easier for a total stranger to see them even under duress. There are some gorgeous masks out there. They could be a statement about your whole personality and identity. (Bonnie)

> I've used cute patterns. . . . I let them all pick and so they all kind of match everybody's personality. I also wanted to make them different so that nobody was accidentally sharing. (Abbie)

> For our work, I wanted cute masks that would transmit the person's personality. . . . I do think that as masks become more a part of our daily lives that people are going to collect them and want to match their outfits and be more indicative of their personality. It's a positive thing. I think that if people can get excited about wearing masks, then that's good for all of us. (Lisa)

Most recently I actually had a request for an entire wedding party. Just around 10 people, but they wanted the masks to match the colors of the wedding. (Amber)

Fashion and function do not have to be mutually exclusive. Regarding masks, an array of fashionable choices could increase usage. A few of our respondents regularly took custom orders. However, most were using the materials they had and therefore not thinking of fashion as a priority but rather a bonus if they had time, materials, and the desire to incorporate users' preferences.

### SELF-EFFICACY DURING CRISES

Respondents expressed that mask making during this time satisfied various personal and communal needs. For some, it was a way to reduce anxiety. For others, there was a sense of civic or moral duty or even patriotism involved. For many, it affirmed that their sewing work is of value, not just a craft. Almost all respondents mentioned that making masks was a useful way they could help others in their community during a time of crisis.

I feel like in any crisis situation, if you can find something you can do, then you should do it. For one, it makes you more sane. . . . I am one who can kind of get in a whirlpool of information, and now I'm about to stroke out because there's all these things. Anything you can control is nice in a situation like this. There is a lot of comfort in just having something you can do. (Tricia)

I must admit, as I made the masks and the people came back, I thoroughly enjoyed saying a few words to them. Staying around the house, it's been hard for me. . . . [My husband and I] both take pride in the fact we have these projects going on. (Edie)

The benefit is personal. It makes me feel productive, like I'm contributing when there's no other way for me to contribute. When we're so worried and afraid of the unknown,

it helps to be busy. My way to deal with stress has always
been frantic activity. (Nancy)

It kind of reminds me of when women would get together
and knit socks for soldiers . . . let's help the war effort. . . .
We're out there with our sewing machines, just like they
did back in World War II, like Rosie the Riveter. . . . It
made me feel that I'm necessary or vital. (Betty Ann)

I've had a lot of issues with being confined to the house,
feeling useful, and so making masks for everyone has really been a way that I could feel like I was contributing and
being able to protect my family. (Abbie)

Just because I'm a crafter does not mean I'm not smart.
And it doesn't mean that I haven't been looking at what's
going to make the best and most effective mask for people
to use at home. . . . These things that for years I've been
told are little things. People look at my sewing as a little
hobby. . . . These things that I have valued for so long.
They do really have value. They have value to the community. They have value beyond even what I thought. And
I feel validated. . . . Confidence in myself—I think it's the
biggest thing I'll take from it. (Mandy)

Making masks was something productive that respondents
could control within an uncontrollable environment. These goals of
empowerment, control, and self-efficacy align with previous literature on response during times of crisis.

### IMPLICATIONS

What went right? Masks already indicated protective actions in the
minds of most Appalachians. Therefore, it wasn't too much of a
mental leap to think of them as protection in the COVID-19 pandemic. Many of our respondents had some prior exposure to mask
usage or had even used them personally for health reasons. Thus,
there was already a degree of comfort related to adoption for these

women, and production was simply the next logical step when mask supplies ran short.

There is a deep connection to self-reliance within Appalachian culture and heritage, as well as a history of communities uniting to support a need. When it came to making masks, these factors combined in a beautiful way. Mask makers displayed self-reliance and efficacy as they researched how to make the best masks and sourced what they could from materials they already had or could get easily. Community members then pitched in for other needs.

Increasing proliferation of technology throughout Appalachia in the past decade enabled mask makers to have a direct connection to the latest information. Promotion also came easily to the mask makers through already established social media channels. In many ways, this eliminated boundaries of communication and information access often associated with health crises. One mask maker even referred to herself as a global citizen, with many others also expressing this idea in other ways.

With some exceptions, many of the women we spoke with were not severely impacted by the current economic recession. They had the ability to do mask-making work to satisfy other personal needs such as self-efficacy, stress relief, altruism, and (socially distanced) socialization. This was especially true for those fully confined to their homes.

The mask makers helped change the dialogue about masks. Most respondents had previously associated masks with those who might have compromised immunity or lived in more polluted areas, but that narrative has now evolved. Even their own wearing of the masks in public helped with normalization of mask usage, and they noted generally receiving far more positive feedback about their efforts than negative. The fact that many name brand clothiers are now making masks also helps in this normalization effort; in this case, fashion can effectively support function. They also mentioned seeing newscasters wearing masks during interviews, which they believe helps to normalize the practice. In short, the more people that wore a mask the better, from both the cultural normalization and public health perspectives.

What went wrong? Information was initially confusing and sometimes contradictory—even when coming from trusted sources such as the CDC and the WHO. It took time for the CDC, a source many used for guidance, to encourage those in nonmedical roles to adopt mask usage, and then it took additional time to encourage cloth mask usage. The sewthecurveflat.com web domain, a resource referenced by one respondent, wasn't even registered until March 21, 2020, more than a week after most of the country began adopting a shelter-in-place protocol. Though major health organizations could have been more prepared and coordinated regarding mask usage protocols and communication efforts, respondents also gave some grace considering how much was initially unknown about the virus and how it was transmitted.

The initial cultural perception in the United States that mask usage was primarily for those already ill or concerned about the spread of germs created tension between mask users and nonusers. The discordant messaging initially put forth by various health and governmental organizations amplified this effect. What began as an uphill cultural battle became a cultural war in some instances, with several mask makers taunted or directly confronted when wearing their masks.

Many of our mask makers were not experiencing immediate financial hardship related to the pandemic and were happy to provide masks for free or for a donation to cover costs. There was unanticipated tension at times when those who needed to sell the masks to make ends meet occasionally noticed friends or others on social media criticizing their sales of the masks. Though this criticism was not the norm, the socioeconomic disparity within the universe of mask makers contributed to some friction.

Many mask makers said they felt overwhelmed by the demand, along with the inability to easily source materials. Some of them wanted better information and greater confidence that what they were doing aided preventative efforts. Even after major health organizations encouraged cloth mask usage, information inconsistency persisted on how masks should be made.

Given all the stories above, what can we take away from this experience moving forward? Mask makers called out several lessons learned. First was a need for better preparation and coordination among major health organizations. Had these protocols been clearer at the onset, particularly regarding mask protocols of when to use a mask and what types should be used in various situations, mask makers believed that there would have been less polarization regarding mask usage.

As for mask creation, makers would have liked a trusted source they could consistently consult for information. A joint effort by some of the major health organizations could fill this need. While many initiatives cited the CDC's stance concerning masks, this information changed several times from March through August, fomenting confusion. A joint health organization effort could also show alignment regarding guidelines and protocols, encouraging unity in the population as well.

Mask makers who felt a unifying factor was needed hoped they would play a role in normalizing the wearing of masks. One respondent mentioned that masks could be considered as a metaphor for kindness, while another stated that they were a visual indicator of a deeply respectful society. Perhaps a campaign promoting mask usage could focus on these character trait goals in the future, when efficacy standards have not yet been proven via extensive study. This could position masks further toward the desired social norm.

Another lesson learned was that social media proved a highly effective way to enable grassroots support for this cause and empower mask makers to promote their efforts. Makers sought support particularly in the form of resources to make masks and the best patterns to use mainly via Facebook and Instagram.

Making a mask helps to connect a person to an action, but it also makes the crisis a reality for people who are removed from COVID-19's effects because they do not know someone who has tested positive or have not yet been exposed to the virus in a way that affects their personal health. It is also an action of solidarity that transcends class, race, physical location, and many other regular divisions.

Mask making and mask usage may become the norm moving forward, or they may become unneeded. Though initial reports regarding mask mandates seemed very promising, we have yet to fully understand the empirical effectiveness of cloth mask usage. Another learned lesson of this time is how swiftly information and recommendations can change best practices. Mask guidelines kept evolving throughout this chapter's publication process, and they likely will continue to do so as more information on efficacy comes to light. As the pandemic winds down, wearing a mask is still an effective way to show support for prevention efforts and heighten awareness of health concerns in the region.

> I am still not 100 percent sure about the importance or
> effectiveness of cloth mask use.... As we've gotten more
> information, even if it's all completely conflicting and
> I still have no idea what this virus actually does or how
> many cases there are, I still have no idea what's going on,
> but I know I don't want any part of it. So if there's any sort
> of barrier where if I have a mask on and you have a mask
> on and that keeps us both from potentially spreading this
> and it doesn't hurt me and it doesn't hurt you, then I feel
> like that's something I can do. (Tricia)

### REFERENCES

1  Kassahunh, P. Elizabethton woman returns to Tri-Cities after being quarantined on a cruise ship that had coronavirus outbreak. WJHL, News Channel 11, March 2, 2020. https://www.wjhl.com/news/local /elizabethton-woman-returns-to-tri-cities-after-being-quarantined -on-a-cruise-ship-that-had-coronavirus-outbreak/.

2  Stobbe, M. More evidence suggests COVID-19 was in US by Christmas 2019. KHOU, June 15, 2021. https://www.khou.com/article/news /health/coronavirus/evidence-suggests-covid-19-in-us-december -2019/507-ffe6209e-e36a-4d5b-83e4-18ed26e0e799.

3  Perreault, M.F., Perreault, G.P. Journalists on COVID-19 journalism: communication ecology of pandemic reporting. *American Behavioral Scientist.* 2021;65(7):887–892. doi.org/10.1177/0002764221992813.

4  McDonald, J. COVID-19 face mask advice, explained. FactCheck, April 6, 2020. https://www.factcheck.org/2020/04/COVID-19-face -mask-advice-explained/.

5 World Health Organization. Advice on the use of masks in the context of COVID-19: interim guidance. WHO, April 6, 2020. https://apps.who.int/iris/handle/10665/331693.

6 Shah, D.T. The COVID-19 crisis: how rural Appalachia is handling the pandemic. *Marshall Journal of Medicine.* 2020;6(2):1.

7 Behringer, B., Friedell, G.H. Appalachia: where place matters in health. *Preventing Chronic Disease.* 2006;3(4):A113.

8 Porter, K., Richards, M. Learning from mom and pop: "making do" in design. *Interdisciplinary Journal of Signage and Wayfinding.* 2019;3(2):29. doi.org/10.15763/issn.2470-9670.2019.v3.i2.a43.

9 Billings, D.B. Insularity, advocacy, and postmodernism in Appalachian studies. *Appalachian Journal.* 2002;29(3):328–332.

10 Welch, W. Self-control, fatalism, and health in Appalachia. *Journal of Appalachian Studies.* 2011;17(1–2):108–122.

11 Durrance, J., Shamblin, W., eds. Appalachian ways: a guide to the historic mountain heart of the East. Washington, DC: US Appalachian Regional Commission, 1976: 31.

12 Keefe, S.E. Mountain identity and the global society in a rural Appalachian county. Institute of Education Sciences, March 5, 2000. https://files.eric.ed.gov/fulltext/ED443646.pdf.

13 Cecelski, E. Rural energy crisis, women's work and family welfare: perspectives and approaches to action. International Labour Organization, No. 992323473402676, June 1984.

14 Seitz, V.R. *Women, Development, and Communities for Empowerment in Appalachia.* Albany: State University of New York Press, 1995.

15 Apostle, E.P., O'Connell, M.E., Vezeau, T.M. Health disparities of coal miners and coal mining communities: the role of occupational health nurses. *AAOHN Journal.* 2011;59(7):311–322.

16 Appalachian Regional Commission. Creating a culture of health in Appalachia. Appalachian Regional Commission, August 2017. https://www.arc.gov/wp-content/uploads/2020/06/Health_Disparities_in_Appalachia_August_2017.pdf.

17 Lane, N.M., Lutz, A.Y., Baker, K., eds. Health care costs and access disparities in Appalachia. Washington, DC: Appalachian Regional Commission, 2012. https://www.arc.gov/report/health-care-costs-and-access-disparities-in-appalachia/.

18 Milkman, R. Women's work and economic crisis: some lessons of the Great Depression. *Review of Radical Political Economics.* 1976;8(1):71–97. doi.org/10.1177/048661347600800107.

19 Kar, S.B., Pascual, C.A., Chickering, K.L. Empowerment of women for health promotion: a meta-analysis. *Social Science & Medicine.* 1999;49(11):1431–1460.

20  Osuch, J.R., Silk, K., Price, C., et al. A historical perspective on breast cancer activism in the United States: from education and support to partnership in scientific research. *Journal of Women's Health.* 2012;21(3):355–362.

21  Lachlan, K.A., Spence, P.R., Lin, X., Najarian, K., Del Greco, M. Social media and crisis management: CERC, search strategies, and Twitter content. *Computers in Human Behavior.* 2016;54:647–652.

22  Reynolds, B., Seeger, M. Crisis and emergency risk communication as an integrative model. *Journal of Health Communication.* 2005;10(1):43–55.

23  Moos, R.H., Schaefer, J.A. Life transitions and crises. In: Moos, R.H., ed. *Coping with Life Crises.* Boston: Springer; 1986:3–28.

24  Spence, P.R., Lachlan, K.A., Burke, J.M. Adjusting to uncertainty: coping strategies among the displaced after Hurricane Katrina. *Sociological Spectrum.* 2007;27(6):653–678.

25  Kiviniemi, M.T., Ram, P.K., Kozlowski, L.T., Smith, K.M. Perceptions of and willingness to engage in public health precautions to prevent 2009 H1N1 influenza transmission. *BMC Public Health.* 2011;11:152. doi.org/10.1186/1471-2458-11-152.

26  Abney, K. "Containing" tuberculosis, perpetuating stigma: the materiality of N95 respirator masks. *Anthropology Southern Africa.* 2018;41(4):270–283.

27  Corrigan, P.W. Mental health stigma as social attribution: implications for research methods and attitude change. *Clinical Psychology: Science and Practice.* 2000;7(1):48–67.

28  Austin, L., Fisher Liu, B., Jin, Y. How audiences seek out crisis information: exploring the social-mediated crisis communication model. *Journal of Applied Communication Research.* 2012;40(2):188–207.

29  Freeman, B., Potente, S., Rock, V., McIver, J. Social media campaigns that make a difference: what can public health learn from the corporate sector and other social change marketers? *Public Health Research and Practice.* 2015;25(2):e2521517.

30  Houston, J.B., Hawthorne, J., Perreault, M.F., et al. (2015). Social media and disasters: a functional framework for social media use in disaster planning, response, and research. *Disasters.* 2015;39(1):1–22.

31  Wendling, C., Radisch, J., Jacobzone, S. The use of social media in risk and crisis communication. OECD Working Papers on Public Governance No. 24. 2013. doi.org/10.1787/19934351.

32  Joachimsthaler, E. The power of social currency. Vivaldi Partners Group. https://vivaldigroup.com/en/2017/10/12/social-currency/. Accessed June 7, 2022.

33 Glaser, B., Strauss, A. *The Discovery of Grounded Theory: Strategies for Qualitative Research.* Chicago: Aldine; 1967.
34 Krippendorff, K. *Content Analysis: An Introduction to Its Methodology.* Thousand Oaks, CA: Sage; 2004.
35 Gordon, S.A. "Boundless possibilities": home sewing and the meanings of women's domestic work in the United States, 1890–1930. *Journal of Women's History.* 2004;16(2):68–91.
36 Lawson, V. Tailoring is a profession, seamstressing is work! Resisting work and reworking gender identities among artisanal garment workers in Quito. *Environment and Planning A.* 1999;31(2):209–227.
37 Pollard, K., Jacobson, L.A. The Appalachian region: a data overview from the 2013–2017 American Community Survey. Appalachian Regional Commission, May 21, 2019. https://www.arc.gov/research/researchreportdetails.asp?REPORT_ID=159.

# 11

## We Already Knew We Were Mortal

*Cancer Patients in the Pandemic*

MONIKA HOLBEIN

*Editor's Note: One of the most poignant experiences pulling these accounts together came from hospice care workers. As the rest of Appalachia (and the world) dealt with mortal fear, hospice patients sighed. Already isolated due to increased infection risks, they watched their comfort medications become hard to get. Relatives who had been their caretakers were unable to provide uplifting social contact, and church or professional drop-off services could no longer deliver the usual round of milk, eggs, and toilet paper as panic buying emptied shops. Hospice patients also found themselves in unique positions to provide comfort to those who usually comforted them, because they heard mortality's whispers in their ears before the pandemic and knew how to practice robust mental health in the shadow of death.*

Cancer and COVID-19 each incite fear in the general population. Exploring how the two interact, especially on how fear of a dual diagnosis affects families and patients, brings out some interesting concepts in health care and in disease stigma. Although long-term effects cannot yet be studied in depth, we can look at the lives of cancer patients and their families in the height of the pandemic.

COVID-19 has increased the worry for death and debility. With information from the initial wave of coronavirus cases indicating that cancer patients, even those in long-term remission, have a higher mortality,[1,2] patients have been appropriately afraid. The psychological burden of not being able to see family members, not going to church, and not socializing with their normal support groups has also been immense. Worries that lurked in the back of patient and family member minds prior to this global health crisis have come to the forefront, for better or worse.

It is common for cancer patients to worry about the mental health of family members caring for them on a daily basis, or at a basic level, even how they are reacting to their loved one's illness. Both patients and families are prone to worry about disease progression, worsening health, and ultimately death. It is normal to be careful around cancer patients in order to avoid transmitting common viruses, and COVID-19 is not like the flu or a common cold. As a result, patients may be delaying care in order to avoid infection situations.[3] On the opposite end of the spectrum, cancer patients are seeking more information, completing advanced directives,[4] and being more involved in their care than previously because the specter of death has increased.

This chapter highlights some of the specific challenges that cancer patients in Appalachia have faced using case scenarios. The patients you meet here have been actively involved in an oncology palliative care clinic for symptom management during the course of their cancer journey; palliative care is for any patient whose illness is not curable and will ultimately end in death. The focus of this specialty is to focus on their symptoms for the duration of their disease course, whether they are still pursuing life-prolonging treatment (with little hope of cure) or have opted to forgo disease-modifying treatment and just focus on their symptoms. Hospice can be involved when patients forgo disease-modifying treatment and have a life expectancy of six months or less as determined by their physician. Hospice focuses on maintaining dignity and treating symptoms aggressively, whether it is pain, nausea, or other distressing symptoms that are affecting a patient's quality of life.

HOWARD: LIFE HASN'T CHANGED MUCH

When I first met Howard, he had just returned from a long stay overseas for work. He had made the difficult decision to return to the United States after he was diagnosed with a hematologic malignancy that would require a transplant. A hematologic malignancy is a cancer of the blood cells. These cells can change and increase in number at an abnormal rate with no real function, leading to cancer.

The lifestyle that he led was not conventional by any means. He lived in the world of concerts and music festivals. He entered the room on his very first visit appointment sporting a skull ring, colorful beads, and a tattered cowboy hat. He openly admitted that smoking marijuana was part of his way of life and that it helped him with his pain and appetite. The pain in his legs was sharp and needlelike, and he just could not get comfortable, even with his medications, prescribed or otherwise obtained. He was agreeable to changing his medications, and his pain was better controlled after we reviewed them and made some adjustments. He also eventually decided that he would rather have synthetic cannabinoid medication instead of continuing with the marijuana.

He was doing well before the COVID-19 pandemic. We had found a delicate balance for his physical symptoms. With the emergence of COVID-19, the clinic made the decision to change the protocol, which had been to see patients monthly for active treatment to assess their symptoms. The hospital and the country as a whole made the push for virtual visits, decreasing in-person patient contact in an effort to reduce the rate of COVID-19 transmission. Howard had the ability to do a video visit.

It was the first time that I was invited into his home. I saw his porch. I saw the river running along his backyard. I saw a person and not a patient at that moment. He showed me around the outside of his home, explaining that he lived here with two friends who cared for him very much. He said that he was doing well. We spoke about how much the world had changed with COVID-19 and social distancing. He asked how my family was doing and how the hospital environment had changed.

When we started to speak about how his life had changed, he said, "Not a lot, doc." He stayed in most days prior to the outbreak for fear that he may get sick because of his compromised immune system. The only difference was that, when his friends went out for food, they wore a mask. They were already doing the other hygiene measures—including handwashing, undressing and showering after being in public, and wiping down groceries to reduce the risk of transmission of any infection—prior to COVID-19. They were also not socializing. The only people that Howard had been in contact with other than health-care workers in the past two years were the two friends that he had been living with, in order to limit the kind of infection opportunities that the whole world was then watching with growing alarm.

Other patients echoed Howard's quiet satisfaction at the realization that other people were now experiencing how they had lived their daily lives for months, even years. Fear of infection had come to the general population, not just people with weak immune systems, and cancer patients found people even reaching out to them for advice on how to keep homes super clean. Before COVID-19, visiting a medically fragile person, one might don a mask or gown, be sure not to have a cold, or observe other kindnesses; and in the back of one's mind, a certain condescension or pity might form. "Hypochondria" or "too much fuss for nothing" might even hover in the thoughts of an uninformed visitor asked to take precautions around a cancer patient. Suddenly, we were all in the same boat.

ANXIETY INCREASING

Cancer Sucks is a well-known nonprofit organization whose mission is to support children and young adults with cancer. There are many other organizations that support cancer patients and further cancer research, but this organization has the most telling title.

Cancer is life changing not only because of the diagnosis and the possible life-limiting consequences but because of its overall impact on daily life. Initially, when patients are told that they may have cancer and need further investigation of blood work, a biopsy, and/

or further imaging, patient anxiety is high.[5] Their appointments may be scheduled in terms of the health-care system norms, which could mean one or two weeks from the time of first suspicion. They spend that time worrying; the effects on health of anxiety over possible cancer diagnoses are well-documented in the literature. (For one example, see "Anxiety and Depression after Cancer Diagnosis: Prevalence Rates by Cancer Type, Gender, and Age," by W. Linden et al., published in 2012 by the *Journal of Affective Disorders*.) Anxiety about future scans may be just as debilitating as that initial diagnosis scan;[6] patients struggle with crippling fear.

Yet this waiting game plays out again and again during the cancer journey: waiting for the next treatment, waiting for the next scan, waiting to complete radiation, waiting for the postchemotherapy symptoms to abate, and many others. Timeliness for treatment can vary greatly across the spectrum, as can awareness of its effects. Anxiety needs a great deal of further investigation on outcomes in lung cancer.[7] Anxiety is also the source of many conversations during visits with patients.

And COVID-19 has increased the waiting "game" to include waiting for family members to be able to visit, waiting to safely go shopping, waiting to go to their appointments without being worried about possible exposure and death, or waiting on family members accompanying them to their appointments to be out of quarantine or to get test results.[8]

LONELINESS DECREASING

COVID-19 has prompted health-care providers to ask cancer patients more about patient interaction with other people. It has been surprising to hear that most patients did not think their lives had changed that much during this pandemic. Cancer patients are constantly worried about being immunocompromised and exposure to any infection that might impact their health. In the Netherlands, the key points of a study exploring the impact of family members on patient health revealed that patients and family members were more at peace (41 percent). Patients felt like they were able to be part of their family's lives again, because everyone was staying home as much as possible. Suddenly it was also possible to see each other, both because of additional time on the part of family members and the limited risks of infection because no one was going anywhere much. This study aims to show that through COVID-19 forcing everyone to practice social distancing, such measures ironically left room for families—and particularly already immunocompromised families, if all were vigilant—to spend more time together. In addition, in-person social circles decreased in size, leaving more qualitative time for families to be together. Even though this was a welcome side effect of COVID-19 social distancing, it did not negate the worries that patients and families had about possible infection and consequences. Patients were still worried about being infected with COVID-19 (50.5 percent) and needing intensive care treatment (65.9 percent). Family members of cancer patients were more worried about infecting their family members (65.9 percent).[9]

CAREGIVER STRAIN

The caregiver burden for patients with chronic illnesses has been increasingly researched in the past 10 years. The burden on caregivers of cancer patients understandably increases with the decrease in patient quality of life.[10] Mental strain and illness is well documented among caregivers, who have a higher incidence of anxiety and depression in comparison to the general population—not least because of financial concerns and burdens related to the illness of their loved one.[11] While caregivers with the political and health-care savvy could sometimes count on in-home professional help from visiting hospice workers or others, stay-at-home orders increased caregiver burnout due to very little outside help and contact.[12]

Navigating the health-care system is challenging even for the health-care literate. Insurance companies, co-pays, prior authorizations, and in-network versus out-of-network providers are all a new language to people who do not work within the system. Navigating this system requires guidance in most cases. Social workers and case managers tend to be the mainstay in this learning process. In cancer centers, they are present during the week to help with patient questions at their appointment and troubleshoot with them for such things as long-term care, in-home help, and who pays for what via insurance and other resources. Since a significant portion of Appalachia's population is Medicare and Medicaid insured and also living rurally without benefit of public transport, patients sometimes need financial support just to get to and from appointments; this means they need help navigating transport voucher programs. They may also need the same for getting their medications: vouchers, Medicaid, Medicare, out of pocket, and insurance can be a quagmire when it comes to prescriptions. In my oncology palliative care clinic, two nurse navigators work closely with the primary oncologist nurse navigators to ensure that patient care includes not just being told what to get but receiving help in getting it. Ours is a novel clinic model that has not been published in the literature to date: we help patients with the storm of information at a time when fear is often reducing their ability to absorb new information. It is not a good time to be stressed when one is fighting for one's life.

The financial burden is a constant worry in cancer patients.[13] The amount of appointments varies, but on average it is at least one every four weeks, many patients having more than that. Each appointment is cause for a co-pay, possible prescription, and travel expenses. Varying grants available depend on financial need, cancer type, and other patient-specific factors; recent grants have been specific to the burden of cancer in the time of COVID-19. Yet the money is limited and again requires a knowledgeable social worker to help the patient to apply for the funds. Most patients are unaware of these funds.

### DELILAH: PRAYING FOR A MIRACLE

Delilah was diagnosed with metastatic disease a few years ago. When she first came, her cancer was causing a significant amount of pain in her abdomen, which improved with one of her first treatments. She and her husband, people of faith, were always hopeful for a cure of her cancer, praying for a miracle.

In the year prior to the start of the pandemic, Delilah had been in and out of the hospital with various infections. There was a visible decline in her overall health. To compound her health troubles, she also had more challenges with her mental health. Her mood was significantly worse. She reported worsening anxiety and depression. She had been seeing a counselor who she said had been ever-so-slightly helpful, and she started seeing a psychiatrist to help with her mental health. During this time, the Delilah's husband mentioned in passing that he noticed she was having trouble thinking at times. All of these changes signaled to the health-care team that it was time to address her end-of-life wishes more consistently and to have a plan in place when she did decline.

Delilah and her husband were given a guide on end of life that was intended to be a conversation starter for them at home with their family members. They took it and agreed to look it over by the next visit. On the next visit, the visit prior to the COVID-19 outbreak, Delilah and her husband became very upset at the mentioning of the guide. This is not an uncommon reaction after patients and families have had time to contemplate a difficult topic. They did not want to speak about these depressing things because she was going to pull through this; faith would get them a miracle, so they did not need to talk about end-of-life care. Then Delilah was hospitalized again for an infection unrelated to COVID-19.

At her visit after that acute hospitalization, her mood changed. She was more peaceful, more resigned. She brought up end-of-life planning. She initiated the conversation. She started speaking while her husband was waiting for her to be done with her appointments because he was unable to accompany her to her appointments. At this point, it became clear to her health-care workers that she was more peaceful with her own death than her husband was, and that the opportunity to speak alone had changed how the conversation could go. With this established, the conversation was paused in order to get her husband to come into the room and join the discussion. After waiting 10 minutes for him to work his way through temperature checks and other screening processes needed to enter the hospital during the pandemic, she again spoke clearly and intentionally. She stated she did not want to be placed on machines. She did not want to have any artificial nutrition. She was OK with God's plan. Her husband cried throughout her speaking. He said repeatedly that he was just hoping for the cancer to go away and that he was so very disappointed that nothing had worked. The past four years of treatment were in vain. She comforted him and told him that she was OK. She completed the Physician Orders for Scope of Treatment form, with the above-mentioned treatments, and in addition she made the decision that her husband could not change her wishes. This was to take away the burden of the decision from him and make it her own.

Delilah died within a week of starting hospice. In the interim, her husband was her primary caretaker. In this case, COVID-19 separating the couple brought an unexpected outcome and perhaps increased peace to the patient.

### HARD CONVERSATIONS, HARD LIVES

Family dynamics are hard. Even on the best of days, there may be disagreements in the most loving families; add in the stress of end-of-life decisions, and these dynamics reach exponential proportions. Appalachia enjoys a long history of multigenerational homes or homesteads, with children less likely to leave the area, so a nuclear family in a cancer patient's life may include parents, children, and grandchildren. A significant portion of the patient population in West Virginia still lives on collective family property.

Prior to COVID-19, West Virginia families were under attack. The opioid epidemic affected every family, some more than others, but no family was left untouched. Grandparents often take on the role of primary caregiver to their grandchildren. The importance of this became very clear during the COVID-19 pandemic. Many of these grandparents are in the at-risk population due to age. When a cancer diagnosis is added to the equation, the patient is at even higher risk. In addition, patients needed to continue with appointments without the security of school to take care of the children while getting treatment. Without a caregiver they can trust, grandparents at times had to choose between their role as a primary caregiver and their own health. Also, because they have seen the effects of painkillers on their addicted children, cancer patient grandparents are often deeply concerned about having opioids in the house. Decreasing patient encounters and the removal of visiting nurses who can be the health-care team's "eyes" within a patient's home delayed action by the health-care team to intervene in unsafe environments. It required weighing the risks and benefits from both perspectives, patient and health-care team, when prescribing opioids. Open conversations and problem solving can help with these dilemmas, but it may not lead to a happy resolution. It may lead to a tenuous balancing act of treating the patient's pain with keeping their family challenges in mind.

The opioid epidemic was perhaps Appalachia's biggest news story prior to COVID-19. It prompted the 2016 "CDC Guideline for Prescribing Opioids for Chronic Pain" to help guide prescribers on safe and effective treatment with the use of opioids.[14] Although the guidelines specifically excluded cancer patients, insurers are not required to make a differentiation, adding financial burden to patient care. West Virginia has specifically started the West Virginia Expert Pain Management Panel to guide practices in the state. These guidelines have been adopted by West Virginia Medicare and Medicaid as steps to approve the use of daily opioid doses above 50 oral morphine equivalents.[15] A recent call has gone out to adopt the CDC guidelines even for opioid prescribing in cancer patients.[16] Knowing that cancer patients are a source of opioids for patients with substance use disorder means that universal precautions cannot be ignored.[17] We need to be mindful of home environments and the unintentional consequences of placing opioids in homes of cancer patients who have a family member struggling with substance use disorder. The balance and understanding that the duo need to achieve for both to feel safe is not to be underestimated. West Virginia is the front-runner in opioid-related overdoses in the United States.[18] Several universities in West Virginia have responded by starting addiction fellowship programs and increasing funding for programs related to substance abuse disorder prevention, management, and harm reduction.

Unfortunately, COVID-19 has now highlighted the importance of continued programming and the disconnects in managing it through a global pandemic. During the preparation and peak of the initial coronavirus wave, treatment centers closed, in-person support meetings were canceled, and other support networks were nonexistent.[19] As of this writing, statistics were still coming in on the results of this, but fatalities appear to have skyrocketed. An interesting article published in 2014 highlights the uniqueness of Appalachia concerning nonmedical opioid use, greater prescription numbers, out-migration of young adults, intense kinship, and economic stressors.[20] Exacerbated by COVID-19 to an extent we cannot yet measure, the social determinants of addiction conditions have highlighted the macabre dance between palliative care, opioid supply in the community, and the responsibility of prescribers. Among the belated yet potentially helpful responses, the judiciary system in West Virginia is modifying court orders for people undergoing a supervised program.[21]

Yet most of the stress is caused not within state systems but in private households. Families with a member who has an active substance use disorder have a unique dynamic in and of themselves.[22] Adding a family with cancer to the equation causes a terrible push and pull. Add in COVID-19, and increased stress is a recipe for more hardship than we can yet understand.

BERNICE: PAIN MANAGEMENT

Bernice has been living with bone cancer for a number of years. Initially she came to the palliative care clinic for continuing and escalating pain treatment for her cancer. The patient at that time was frustrated that she was not able to do the things that she had loved to do prior to her cancer diagnosis. The biggest frustration was that she was unable to cook anymore without significant pain. After a few visits, she also confided that she was constantly worried about the cancer worsening. Every time that she had a little more pain, her worry would be so great that she had more cancer, until she was able to have her next imaging study. After exhausting oral pain medications, she was referred to the interventional pain clinic for a possible pain pump. The patient reacted well to the pain pump trial and was set to have one inserted at the end of March 2020. This was delayed due to COVID-19.

The cycle of worry was impacting her life just as greatly as the pain from her cancer. She lived in an area with no mental health professionals, and the drive to the cancer center was more than an hour, so she was unable to come for weekly psychotherapy sessions. She did, however, start seeing a psychiatrist who was able to help her once a month. That also stopped during the pandemic, since broadband in her region could not support virtual meetings.

When COVID-19 first began to impact daily life, she had an imaging study because of increasing pain. When asked more closely, the patient stated that the pain was not constant and did not have any correlation to activity or other things that she did in her day. The imaging study showed that she had a vertebral fracture. The patient was hopeful that an increase in her oral pain medications would help with the pain, but they did not. She was then offered a referral to an interventional physician for possible kyphoplasty (vertebra cementing), which he was happy to do for her. The date and the time had been approved for April 2020, but when the patient was called, she declined intervention. She did not want to come to the hospital during COVID-19 and risk infection. Also, she just really wanted to wait for the pain pump, because she hoped that this would make the pain go away.

IMPACTS OF THE OPIOID CRISIS IN PALLIATIVE CARE

Over the past few years, the world of oncology, and with it the world of palliative care, has changed in so many ways. Gone are the days when we were able to treat pain symptoms with pharmaceuticals alone. Because of the opioid crisis, patients are now being referred to alternatives including physical therapy, occupational therapy, and other longer-term directed treatments for their overall health. Pain medication whenever possible is reserved for end-of-life care. We must be part of opioid stewardship moving forward to ensure that there are medications available to treat symptoms at the end of life aggressively. Also, in the United States, and more specifically in Appalachia, cancer patient prescribers must be diligent in monitoring patients. The number-one way in which people become addicted to nonprescribed painkillers is through access via a patient. The bottle is on a shelf, and the experimental teen wishes to be the hit of a party—or, in pandemic days, to reduce the stress of online school and reduced friend access.

As mentioned earlier, prior to the emergence of COVID-19 patients were on average seen in person every four weeks for close follow-up; most of these appointments combined with their chemotherapy or immunotherapy infusions to decrease the trips to the cancer center. At the beginning of the pandemic, confusion reigned on how to proceed, especially without reimbursement of telemedicine visits. That was the regulation prior to COVID-19. There was much discussion on how to safely continue to treat patients while not losing them to follow-up. The first thought was to focus on the patients who did not have other appointments in the cancer center and do an informal risk stratification to determine which patients could be seen three months later. The patients would need to take the initiative to call in for medication refills. The phone call would be returned, and the patient would have a phone visit to discuss the use and effectiveness of their current regimen. Patients who had in-person treatment in the cancer center would continue to be seen on a regular basis, without the initial assessment by the nurse clinician.

The difficulty in this initial strategy was that the patients could not be seen in person to assess their movement, posture, and other things that the patients do not readily mention without prompting. The other challenge was ensuring that patients who were on long-term opioids would be able to fill them without running out because they called in for refills too late.

With the Centers for Medicare and Medicaid Services (CMS) response to the pandemic allowing telehealth visits to be reimbursed, flexibility increased to follow patients more closely and continue the

highest safest quality care. Prior to this response, there were very specific guidelines for reimbursement from video visits, and telephone
visits were not reimbursable. Video visits would be reimbursed at the
same rate as in-person visits during the COVID-19 pandemic.
While this was good news, the challenge within rural Appalachia was soon evident. The internet is not reliable here, and some
homes lack access to broadband completely. Even when patients
were able to initiate a video visit, the internet speed prevented the
connection, or the connection was too slow to work well enough for
a visit, constantly freezing or needing a reboot. If you want to see
a frustrated physician, watch one who budgeted time for multiple
appointments and has to cancel half of them due to slow internet
speeds. Even within a 20-minute driving radius of Morgantown,
several neighborhoods lack internet access other than by satellite,
which is unreliable at best. This burden falls primarily on communities of color and on low-income communities.

On a positive side, video visits do allow for caregivers to be present during the interview to help with the history and to interject
any important points. Patient family members can be an important
part of any decision-making process when the online appointment
works. Without their presence, patients rarely make final decisions
about altering or forgoing further treatment.

Bernice's situation, for instance, needed more than a telehealth
visit could provide. She required an in-person appointment to further evaluate and treat her increasing pain.

After the difficulty with video visits was recognized by legislators, CMS then approved telephone visits to be reimbursed at
the higher rate. The pandemic did cause legislators to move more
swiftly than normal, also a good thing. With both virtual visit types
(phone or online), there is no way to obtain samples such as a urine
drug screen, or even the all-important visual clues that practitioners
who trained during the opioid crisis know almost instinctively. Telephone visits continue to be suboptimal for patient care, as there is
no visual component to the exam/interview, but when the internet
is not up to the job, they are better than nothing. A large amount

of trust must be placed into the patient's given history when visual clues disappear, and of course prescribing in these "blind" moments is not something anyone wanted to contemplate.

Trying to chip away at the opioid epidemic is important, but the most important reason for the in-person frequent follow-up is to catch the patient before they fall—meaning to prevent morbidity and mortality. The best predictors of mortality are the observable losses (or gains) of milestones in daily activity and self-care that patients experience. With virtual visits, we are unable to assess their functional status regularly. This delays interventions and possible changes in overall treatment. It means those going into decline may reach a crisis point before being diagnosed, and those improving may not have a concomitant reduction in medication.

In-person visits during COVID-19 had multiple stressors: the absence of caregivers who had gone to work in the heart of the pandemic crisis or who had decided to take time away during the crisis. Some hospital systems, stressed economically because of patient decisions to put off routine care, furloughed providers—a concept that sends the mind reeling. During a global pandemic, so few people went to the hospital that they were forced to reduce staff? Welcome to the strange world of health-care supply and demand. Patient decisions should be honored, as in the case of Bernice, who opted for a pain pump over vertebrate repair because of her fear of COVID-19.

As face-to-face patient encounters became more possible, summer giving way to autumn 2020, even then new challenges arose in palliative care. Caregivers could not accompany patients; previously, they had been there not only to lend support but as an active part of the conversation about end-of-life care for their loved ones and as an extra set of listening ears. As mentioned before, anxiety impedes cognitive ability to process new information. Patients may not retain all of the information given to them or may at times remember the conversation inaccurately. Caregivers were a safeguard against lost or misunderstood information. They were also a hand to hold during lengthy treatments or long days moving through hospitals.

When they were not allowed such support (with a few exceptions for those cognitively impaired or entering end-of-life decisions), patients given the option to return to monthly visits would forgo treatment or visits because they did not wish to attend without their caregiver. Although it is for the benefit of others to reduce the transmission of possible COVID-19, it proved significantly stressful in the cancer population. This does indicate that at times a video visit may be the right form of visit for the patient if not receiving active cancer treatment.

### WALTER: QUALITY OF LIFE

Walter's cancer, according to conventional knowledge, should have taken his life years ago. Cancer treatments have radically changed, making some cancer types more of a chronic illness than an immediately life-limiting illness. The first contact the palliative care physician had with him was in the hospital while he was confused and diagnosed with pneumonia. Palliative care is focused on the patient's illness experience and how to improve it with the patient's goals in mind. Walter's focus was to live the longest life possible; this meant that his time was more important than the quality of his life. The radical treatment advances that oncology makes on a yearly basis continue to be a learning experience for all non-oncologists, doctors, nurses, and patients alike.

During his last four years, the patient was able to spend time with his grandchildren, who were the driving force for his continued treatment, and to spend time with the rest of his family. He enjoyed time fishing and shooting his slingshot. He enjoyed life with the ongoing chemotherapy and the other symptomatic treatments. He lived with a family member who was devoted to him and his goals, even though they were not always aligned with those of his other family members.

The second week of the COVID-19 social distancing order, the family member called and stated that she was not coming to his treatments, as she did not want to get COVID-19. She was also worried about him because he was spending 24 hours a day in bed and picking and choosing which medications to take. This was in line with his ornery personality. He did take a phone call from the palliative care physician to speak about possible hospice involvement, stating that he would think about it. The next day on follow-up, he did not take the call and told his family member to say that he was not interested. The family member was so tearful and was worried about the future because she was struggling to take care of him. She was unable to call their support system to come and help because of COVID-19. The patient and his caregiver were alone in the crisis, except for occasional home health aides coming to the home. Five days before he died, hospice was finally allowed to come into the home to help him and his family.

### FAMILY, FAITH, AND PAST EXPERIENCES

The *New York Times* article "The Time for 'the' Talk Is Now" (May 19, 2020) really embodies the thought process that needs to be adopted by patients and physicians alike. End-of-life care is not a one-size-fits-all affair. Decisions are multifaceted. The big influencing factors are family, faith, and past experiences. These can also be looked at in their larger context: decision maker–related criteria, decision-specific criteria, and contextual factors.[23] The uncertainty surrounding COVID-19 infections has caused many to rethink putting off writing down their thoughts and wishes. This is always best done with the guidance of a physician who knows the patient well, and it is an ongoing conversation rather than one written in stone. End-of-life wishes change over time.

For example, before I had children, my end-of-life wishes were clear: if I could not participate in life, including my hobbies and my profession as a physician, I was okay with less aggressive treatment. As soon as I became a mother, this changed to aggressive treatment until the day that I proved unable to observe my children's growth and happiness. This is just one example of how end-of-life wishes (or *living wishes,* as we prefer to call them) are malleable. To this end, the best living wills are the ones written thoughtfully by the patient, with clear expectations of what they accept as their livable life. Unfortunately, these living wills are not the norm, at least not pre-COVID-19. The norm is a form document that states if a doctor deems that the patient is at the end of life, the patient would like to be made comfortable and not continue aggressive treatment.

When we take a closer look at the three influencing factors for medical decision-making mentioned above, family comes first in every sense. The disproportionate number of grandparents raising their grandchildren due to the substance abuse crisis has put a greater burden on the grandparents to continue to stay alive to care for their grandchildren. Their own children continue to come in and out of their lives at undetermined intervals, living with them or just visiting. This complicates how a grandparent cancer patient might make life-wish decisions. Even though a medical power of attorney may have been designated by the patient, this does not exclude them from involving their family in the process as time goes on.[24]

In addition, if the patient's wishes were not delineated well previously, verbally or in a well-written document, this can lead to a significant amount of discussion and at times challenges in communication—particularly when estranged or angry children in active drug use become involved. COVID-19 added another level of complexity to this already tense situation.

COVID-19 is a sudden illness with what can be a prolonged course of treatment and recovery if severe. There have been cases of young, healthy people dying of COVID-19 who most likely have not had discussions with their families about medical decision-making or about their medical power of attorney. People under 30 rarely thought about such things prior to the pandemic. Grandparents who fear dying and leaving their grandchildren with irresponsible parents often make decisions that those parents challenge. If such things are not written down in a formal way, these challenges might prove successful. The pandemic increased awareness of this among people of all ages.

Family dynamics influence our decisions as providers about what the perceived role of the patient is within the family, both from a patient perspective and a family perspective. As mentioned, the patient may see their role as vital to the rest of the family members' well-being and livelihood. The family may view the patient as the matriarch or patriarch without whom they are not able to function. End-of-life care was hard enough to discuss in situations where substance abuse and age were the driving factors; add in potential exposure to COVID-19 when the mother of the children comes to visit, unaware she is infected, and you can see the stress under which grandparents live.

Faith in Appalachia largely consists of Christianity in various forms. Identifying as Christian does not mean a single type of decision-making process; asking patients and family members how their faith influences their medical decision-making process is helpful, and sometimes the faith group itself can be an unexpected ally.[25] As an example, for decades, Catholics tended to believe that it was a sin to withhold nutrition from their family members. The Catholic Church finally took a stance on this: if the artificial nutrition will not prolong life in a meaningful way, then it is okay to withhold it.

When we think about faith-based medical decision-making, we often think of the attitude of Delilah: hoping for a miracle or "God is in charge." These are statements that physicians need to follow up with a question to fully understand their meaning. There is quite a bit of literature regarding hoping for a miracle or trusting in a higher power.[26] Yet when we ask more specifically about what a miracle might entail, we may be surprised by the answer.[27] Sometimes it is as simple as living long enough to be at a wedding or birth, not the sudden removal of all illness. Chaplains may help explore these subtleties more.[28] Physicians in palliative care have learned not to take "miracle" as having a specific meaning, and it is my observation that physicians working with COVID-19 patients are discovering the same.

Past experiences are not to be discounted. A patient with chronic obstructive pulmonary disease that has been on a ventilator in the past and proves able to come off of the ventilator may be more amenable to trying such intervention again. Also, a patient who has had successful CPR is more likely to say that they would like this to be done again. On the flip side, this holds true with patients who have had bad experiences with family members. For example, a patient whose family member died quickly and poorly after being diagnosed with lung cancer may be more hesitant to try chemotherapy for fear of dying quickly even with interventions. In addition, healthcare experiences as a whole and involvement in one's care can also speak to future care. If a patient has typically avoided going to the doctor, coming to the office for weekly visits may not be what they are able or willing to do. COVID-19 complicated this because the experiences came fast, and the virus was novel. People made false comparisons to pneumonia, flu, even bronchitis, assuming they had time to make any comparisons at all. In the cancer population, exposure to COVID-19 was often discovered by acute distress, not symptoms. Using past experiences in a new situation is hit or miss.

Lastly, oncologists and primary care physicians of cancer patients always remember that no decision is a decision in and of itself. The patient may say that they would rather have their family make the decision for them or leave that unsaid. In some cultures, adult children may make decisions for their parents if they feel the diagnosis would overwhelm them.[29] Kicking the can down the road is in and of itself a decision. We don't push on these thin walls of dignity. Will this result in a good death? Maybe it will, for the patient.

Hospice in COVID-19 has been challenging. Many questions have arisen on how to keep patients and health-care workers safe. Patients may opt not to start hospice services until a later date to decrease the amount of people coming in and out of their homes. Inpatient hospice services may not be utilized because family members worry about not seeing their loved one again.[30] Hospice workers still, in fall 2020, did not have adequate personal protective equipment, although 2021 improved slowly.

Overall, COVID-19 exacerbated existing crisis issues in Appalachia more than created new ones. It again brought the opioid epidemic to the fore, and perhaps highlighted what people tend to forget: that it impacts all aspects of society. Access to care even with the option of telehealth continues to be an issue with poor connectivity. Perhaps the only new challenge was that our family-centric society struggled with the loss of interaction with each other.

Much can be learned from the challenges that COVID-19 brought to our region. There is room for growth and improvement. Protocols continue to evolve. Medicine is also changing at an ever-increasing pace, trying to outpace the effects of COVID-19 and keep it from pushing us backwards, erasing the progress made on the substance abuse crisis.

One thing COVID-19 could not change, however: Appalachians have always been and always will be a connected, resilient people. The pandemic did not take that away from us.

## REFERENCES

1 Zhang, H., Wang, L., Chen, Y., et al. Outcomes of novel coronavirus disease 2019 (COVID-19) infection in 107 patients with cancer from Wuhan, China. *Cancer.* 2020;126:4023–4031. doi:10.1002/cncr.33042.

2 Li, Qiubai, Chen, L., Li, Qin, et al. Cancer increases risk of in-hospital death from COVID-19 in persons <65 years and those not in complete remission. *Leukemia.* 2020;34(9):2384–2391. doi:10.1038/s41375-020-0986-7.

3 Masroor, S. Collateral damage of COVID-19 pandemic: delayed medical care. *Journal of Cardiac Surgery.* 2020;35:1345–1347. doi:10.1111/jocs.14638.

4 Portz, J.D., Brungardt, A., Shandbhag, P, Staton, E. Advance care planning among users of a patient portal during the COVID-19 pandemic: retrospective observational study. *Journal of Medical Internet Research.* 2020;22(8):e21385. doi:10.2196/21385.

5 Iwamitsu, Y., Shimoda, K., Abe, H., Tani, T., Okawa, M., Buck, R. Anxiety, emotional suppression, and psychological distress before and after breast cancer diagnosis. *Psychosomatics.* 2005;46(1):19–24. doi: 10.1176/appi.psy.46.1.19.

6 Bauml, J.M., Troxel, A., Epperson, C.N., et al. Scan-associated distress in lung cancer: quantifying the impact of "scanxiety." *Lung Cancer.* 2016;100:110–113. doi: 10.1016/j.lungcan.2016.08.002.

7 Olsson, J.K., Schultz, E.M., Gould, M.K. Timeliness of care in patients with lung cancer: a systematic review. *Thorax.* 2009;64(9):749–756. doi:10.1136/thx.2008.109330.

8 Storino, C.B., Watson, J.C., Sanchez, W., et al. Revamping outpatient care for patients without COVID-19. *Mayo Clinic Proceedings.* 2020;95(9):S44–S46. doi.org/10.1016/j.mayocp.2020.06.010.

9 Schellekens, M.P., Van Der Lee, M.L. Loneliness and belonging: exploring experiences with the COVID-19 pandemic in psycho-oncology. *Psycho-oncology.* 2020;29(9):1399–1401. doi:10.1002/pon.5459.

10  Borges, E.L., Franceschini, J., Costa, L.H.D., et al. Family caregiver burden: the burden of caring for lung cancer patients according to the cancer stage and patient quality of life. *Jornal Brasileiro de Pneumologia*. 2017;43(1):18–23. doi: 10.1590/S1806-37562016000000177.

11  Williams, A.L., McCorkle, R. Cancer family caregivers during the palliative, hospice, and bereavement phases: a review of the descriptive psychosocial literature. *Palliative & Supportive Care*. 2011;9(3):315–325. doi:10.1017/S1478951511000265.

12  Park, S.S. Caregivers' mental health and somatic symptoms during COVID-19. *Journals of Gerontology: Series B*. 2020;76(4):e235–e240. doi:10.1093/geronb/gbaa121.

13  Amir, Z., Wilson, K., Hennings, J., Young, A. The meaning of cancer: implications for family finances and consequent impact on lifestyle, activities, roles and relationships. *Psycho-oncology*. 2012;21(11):1167–1174. doi: 10.1002/pon.2021.

14  Dowell, D., Haegerich, T.M., Chou, R. CDC guideline for prescribing opioids for chronic pain—United States. *Morbidity and Mortality Weekly Report*. 2016;65(RR-1):1–49.

15  Safe & effective management of pain guidelines. Semp Gudelines. https://www.sempguidelines.org. Accessed June 9, 2022.

16  Arthur, J., Bruera, E. Balancing opioid analgesia with the risk of nonmedical opioid use in patients with cancer. *Nature Reviews Clinical Oncology*. 2019;16(4):213–226. doi:10.1038/s41571-018-0143-7.

17  Manchikanti, L., Prescription drug abuse: what is being done to address this new drug epidemic? Testimony before the Subcommittee on Criminal Justice, Drug Policy and Human Resources. *Pain Physician* 2006;9(4):287–321. https://pubmed.ncbi.nlm.nih.gov/17066115/.

18  Scholl, L., Seth, P., Kariisa, M., Wilson, N., Baldwin, G. Drug and opioid-involved overdose deaths—United States, 2013–2017. *Morbidity and Mortality Weekly Report*. 2019;67(5152):1419–1427. doi:10.15585/mmwr.mm675152e1.

19  Cyders, M.A., Ladd, K.L., Fry, M.S. People with substance use disorders face greater challenges during the COVID-19 pandemic. The Conversation, 2020. https://theconversation.com/people-with -substance-use-disorders-face-greater-challenges-during-the-covid -19-pandemic-137476.

20  Keyes, K.M., Cerdá, M., Brady, J.E., Havens, J.R., Galea, S. Understanding the rural-urban differences in nonmedical prescription opioid use and abuse in the United States. *American Journal of Public Health*. 2014;104(2):e52–e59. doi:10.2105/ajph.2013.301709.

21  Hrdinova, J., Berman, D.A., Pauley, M., Ridgway, D. Documenting the challenges (and documents) as Ohio courts respond to COVID-19. *Ohio State Public Law Working Paper*, 2020.

22  Kumpfer, K.L., Alvarado, R., Whiteside, H.O. Family-based inter-
    ventions for substance use and misuse prevention. *Substance Use &
    Misuse* 2003;38(11–13):1759–1787. doi:10.1081/JA-120024240.
23  Glatzer, M., Panje, C.M., Sirén, C., Cihoric, N., Putora, P.M. De-
    cision making criteria in oncology. *Oncology.* 2020;98(6):370–378.
    doi:10.1159/000492272.
24  Sudore, R.L. Preparing surrogates for complex decision mak-
    ing: the often neglected piece of the advance care planning equa-
    tion. *JAMA Internal Medicine.* 2019;179(2):268–269. doi:10.1001/
    jamainternmed.2018.5280.
25  Khalid, K., Ku Md Saad, S., Abd Ghani, N.A., Mohamed Abdul Kad-
    her, A.N. Religious and cultural challenges in paediatrics palliative
    care: A review of literature. *Pediatric Hematology Oncology Journal.*
    2019;4(3):67–73. doi:10.1016/j.phoj.2019.11.001.
26  Bibler, T.M., Stahl, D., Fantus, S., Lion, A., Brothers, K.B. A process-
    based approach to responding to parents or guardians who hope
    for a miracle. *Pediatrics.* 2020;145(3):e2019–2319. doi:10.1542/
    peds.2019–2319.
27  George, L.S., Balboni, T.A., Maciejewski, P.K., Epstein, A.S., Priger-
    son, H.G. "My doctor says the cancer is worse, but I believe in
    miracles"—when religious belief in miracles diminishes the impact
    of news of cancer progression on prognostic understanding change.
    *Cancer.* 2020;126(4):832–839. doi:10.1002/cncr.32575.
28  Torke, A.M., Fitchett, G., Maiko, S., et al. The association of surrogate
    decision makers' religious and spiritual beliefs with end-of-life deci-
    sions. *Journal of Pain and Symptom Management* 2020;59(2):261–269.
    doi:10.1016/j.jpainsymman.2019.09.006.
29  Mori, M., Morita, T. End-of-life decision-making in Asia: a need for
    in-depth cultural consideration. *Palliative Medicine,* January 2020.
    doi:10.1177/0269216319896932.
30  Mercadante, S. The clash between palliative care and COVID-19.
    *Supportive Care in Cancer.* 2020;28(12):5593–5595. doi:10.1007/
    s00520-020-05680-x.

# 12

## Nursing While Black

SOJOURNER NIGHTINGALE

*Editor's Note: As in the chapter on cancer patients, the pandemic caused a reckoning in many lives, an assessment of attitudes and perhaps adjustments. Nationally, George Floyd's videotaped murder during the summer of 2020 became the lightning rod coalescing calls for racial reckonings. Has the bill come due to the United States on racial inequality? We've been here before, say Black authors weary with deferred hope. Health-care heroes? The feel-good narrative of pulling together during the pandemic wears thin as accounts like this chapter emerge. If setting aside prejudices during a global crisis cannot happen at local levels, what does this say about the future of racial justice in Appalachia? Note particularly how ignored messages about public health and safety compare to messages about racial reckoning, and why. What is your role in this reckoning?*

I grew up in an area in which I was a minority. Blacks are considered statistically insignificant in my town. Most of my childhood was an uphill battle with the education system, so my life has been about fighting the odds. I dreamed of being a nurse since childhood and turned that into reality when it came time to go to college. Mostly that was because of relatives who died when I was in high school. I felt like they would still be alive had they had a good nurse. I was hoping to bring a Black voice and perspective into health care in the Appalachian region.

I am the only Black nurse in my unit. There are other Black nurses in the system, but we don't work together. Mostly we work as the only Black person on our team, but we know each other because of our support network. The staff in my team is split between middle-aged White women, younger White women, and a few White men.

Growing up in this area of Appalachia, as a survival mechanism I learned how to make White southerners feel comfortable around me. When I was younger, it was a security blanket I wanted to be under. Now that I am older, I realize that I became tokenized—turned into "the Good Negro" stereotype that White people wanted me to be. I still remember comments, as far back as middle school, about how I was "not like the other ones." Do we become our choices, or can we bust back out of them?

Long before COVID, when I had my first Black patient a few months after starting work, another nurse went into the room and helped her use the bedpan. When she came out, she said, "Make sure you don't act like that one if you're ever here." I then realized that if I were to have a medical emergency, I would still face bias from the very people I work alongside. Perhaps that comment from my colleague was when I truly started to question how well the Black community in my area is treated. Or maybe it started in elementary school, when the teachers told me I couldn't be a nurse.

On my weekend off at the beginning of 2020, a young Black patient died. Nobody knew quite what happened, when I got back and asked. They said his condition deteriorated rapidly. I still wonder if his complaints were ignored.

Not long after, two patients were admitted on the same night. The first was a young White man in boots and a T-shirt; he weighed over 200 pounds. The other was a 40-something Black man in business dress, weak and skinny. The charge nurse had the White man's dip (tobacco) and a knife put in the dresser drawer by his bed so he could reach them easily. She confiscated the Black man's wallet, cigarettes, and knife.

I took care of another Black patient later that same week. His family thanked me and told me they were proud of me and encouraged me to go as far as I can in my profession. A nurse who overheard them was offended by that conversation. She said she felt that my success should be remarked on separately from my Blackness; to put them together was somehow a form of racist comment. That nurse is not a person who shares the all-too-familiar ideology of constant wrongdoing by a person of color, so it startled me that she couldn't understand. Well, maybe not startled me; maybe the right word is *disappointed*?

I started thinking about suggesting a mandatory refresher course for seasoned nurses after that incident. But when you get a group of rural Appalachian nurses together, cultural sensitivity inevitably swings toward themselves, how Appalachians are stereotyped and misunderstood and portrayed as dumb by the media, and so on. Would there be any point in trying to make the experiences of Black staff visible to them?

There were always plenty of things to be wary of, and to be aware of, at work. Then one day in March, everything changed—for the worse. *COVID-19* became the most common word used in my hospital. People were uncertain about the seriousness of it. My kids came home from school, and we found out literally overnight that they would not be returning for a couple of weeks—no warning. I thought the response was being blown out of proportion until I found myself watching the statistics of other countries. Nope, not overblown. We were in for it.

Being the medical worker in my family, I was immediately bombarded with calls and concerns, even before I could assess the threat we were under. Relatives I did not closely associate with started to text me for updates. My nearby relatives and friends warned me not to trust anything my job might give me for prevention. It wouldn't work, they meant. As in, Black nurses wouldn't be the priority recipients of good personal protective equipment (PPE).

They were right. I had varying degrees of support, but it didn't come from my employer, who refused to do a respirator fit test on me. The test was to fit an individual's face to the N95 masks that had become the gold standard for COVID patient care. Every other nurse in my unit was tested. No explanation was ever given for why I wasn't. (If you were about to ask, "Why didn't you complain to HR?" I'll pause and give you some time to think about why a Black employee would not do that—especially when she had witnessed a friend in another unit get fired for insubordination.) I mentioned this to someone connected with a local nonprofit, which then sent me one N95, two cloth masks, and a surgical cap in the mail.

Tensions were high in my household. My husband worried about me. We both worried about our kids. My oldest daughter was old enough to understand what was going on, and she worried about me, which made me worry about her even more.

The visitor policy changed at my hospital. At first, we joked about getting to kick out annoying relatives, but then reality set in. I felt like I was walking the green mile when clocking in. I came down a long, empty, shiny hallway. The masks, cloth or surgical, were a nuisance, but a necessary evil. At first, we would attempt to smile at each other under them, but as time went on, we didn't as often. Work hours were reduced while elective procedures were canceled. I thought it would result in more family time, but I was more drained on my abbreviated schedule than I was when working long hours. Being on high alert is exhausting.

Social media made it worse. Anti-vaxxers were the first I saw to post conspiracy theories about "them" creating a vaccine for population control and advising against it. Even intellectuals I respected were posting unfounded information about the lockdowns and the need for us all to wear masks.

My cousin up north did not believe COVID-19 was deadly until she lost a friend to it. She still blames the hospital instead of the virus. She swears they killed her friend and advised others not to go to the hospital if they got sick. There were scriptures, mostly from the book of Revelation, being shared. I started to hear about 5G towers and microchips.

I had relatives asking me if I was required to get any type of shot to keep my job. I was asked if I was required to put COVID as the cause of death on death certificates to get my hospital money, another fun rumor floating around on Facebook and other places. I had never had someone question my ethics personally before, but I somehow became a beacon overnight without asking to be; no one from the Black or White communities, no strangers in stores or family members online, hesitated to ask questions ranging from insensitive to downright accusatory. Did we really have COVID patients in our hospital, or was it all a big hoax? How many doctors had COVID but were still working? The questions were all over the place. Boundaries didn't exist and I got exhausted trying to create them.

Black people are all too familiar with conversations that can turn in an instant. One day when we were at the station together just before going into patient rooms, a coworker came out with how Breonna Taylor shouldn't have been dating a drug dealer, so it was her fault she got shot. The father of that coworker's child was in prison for drug offenses.

I called her on trashing Breonna's reputation but left that second part alone. Walk the line, and be prepared for owning the callout beyond that shift. Best case: your coworker stops talking to you. Worse case: your coworker tells all the other team members to stop talking to you. Worst possible case: your coworker finds a way to get human resources involved. It may be her problem, but you will wear it, and that is exhausting. Yet it is important. Who will speak if I don't? That's one reason Black people are tired all the time. And why we don't try to explain why we're tired all the time. We need to conserve energy for the times when we have to call out what we're hearing, or seeing, and for the aftermath of doing so.

I was uncertain about the future and about going out in public. I bought my food two weeks at a time and ordered a few subscription boxes to help. I felt like Typhoid Mary when I ran errands. People would avoid me when they saw me in scrubs. This experience was surreal. I kept seeing signs and promotions calling me a hero, but I did not feel like one with the dirty looks and rude comments at the grocery store. They didn't call me "hero" there. The words were different.

I started to see unsourced stories of Black people being given experimental treatments and getting worse and/or dying. One side of my family was arguing reasons not to lock down because we did not need higher unemployment. The other side of my family was arguing to stay home unless absolutely necessary and that reopening hair salons and churches was just a sneaky way to draw out Black people.

My brain was constantly in motion. I checked every beep on my phone, worried about relatives, and subscribed to every applicable website looking for news and updates. I wondered if I would get a stimulus check. I thought about my relatives whose rent would not even be covered by that payment. I wanted to advise them, but I had no idea what to tell them. That was a common theme as relatives kept asking for medical advice, behavioral advice, and insights on which parts of the pandemic were aimed at Black people specifically. Was it safe to go to the hospital if they got sick?

I have seen young people die from this virus. I have seen elderly people survive it. I know that my community, my Black community, gets hit harder during any type of crisis. I wondered how my loved ones would be treated at their local facilities, as well as the one I work for, if they had to go in for care. I didn't have an easy answer for any questions.

Though disparities hit us in a different way, our country and the entire world were all in trouble. A meme started circling on Facebook about canoes and yachts trying to weather the same storm. We did not know what to expect in our quiet corner of rural living, how hard we were going to be hit as a hospital, or how hard it was going to hit us as individuals. April, May, June, July passed with fewer cases than layoffs and furloughs. August was hot. September, the little needles of infection pockets started to coalesce. October, November, December, January, we were on fire. We had wanted to believe it was hype, but then we started to see it come closer. Mobile morgue trucks rolled up in our flagship hospital parking lot. That freaked us all out. That kind of thing just didn't happen here.

I started smelling my soap every morning when I returned home from work, to help me feel safe. That is, until the day I had a dry cough and fatigue. I told my employee health office about my symptoms. I had to get swabbed, but my employer—the biggest regional health-care system in the area—couldn't do it. I called three differ-ent facilities trying to get tested, and they each told me something different—except, they each told me no in the end.

I wondered if my Black voice on the phone made them treat me as though I weren't a health-care worker. So for the next place I called, I said over and over again that I was a health-care worker and needed a rapid test. I was finally able to get an appointment the next day. Yay, but I was angry that I had to exhaust myself to get what other health-care workers got the first time they asked.

At the testing site, I asked the lady if she'd been told that I needed a rapid test, and she told me it was rapid and swabbed me. I did not want to correct her, but what she did was not the way that we were trained to do the swab. She did not go far enough at all, just about guaranteeing it would come back negative. She was also not courte-ous and complained about being late for lunch. I went home scared, sick, and awaiting results. I called the facility and asked how long the results would be and they said it would be back in a few hours. I finally was told three days later that I was negative. My oxygen would drop into the mid-80s when I moved a certain way (it should be in the mid to high 90s), yet they never confirmed that I had it.

I returned to work. I couldn't stay home because the test was neg-ative. I felt like a leper. I was already anxious, walking down the shiny, empty hallways with hot air hitting my face from patient rooms. I did not feel comfortable being near my patients, yet they were longing for contact with other people because of the visiting restrictions. I wanted to hold their hands, but knew I should not. Negative or not, every-thing said that I had COVID. She had tested me wrong. I was still early enough to be contagious—less than seven days.

Throughout the pandemic, every time a code was called, my heart sank. Eager new grads who watch too many medical dramas learn quickly that codes are nothing like the shows portray. COVID diagnosis codes were especially gut wrenching. A limited number of people were allowed in at a time. There would only be one person in the room to relieve the other from compressions. We had to don PPE before we entered the room, and each time I would wonder if the delay decreased their chances of survival. At a time when town halls, restaurants, and social media posts called us heroes, our infection control training, the CDC, and our own better judgment told us not to be a hero and protect ourselves first.

There was also my mask problem. I was the only nurse not given an N95 mask for going into coding patient rooms—the rooms of people who were dying of COVID. The one from the charity lasted more than a week. After that, four times I ran into a coding room without a mask. After the second code, I spoke to my nurse manager. She was confused at first, but when she realized what was happening, she spoke to her superiors. In the end, silence came from that part of the hospital, but the house supervisor brought me an N95 and told me to write my name on the inside of it and keep it with me at all times. She did not offer an explanation for why I hadn't had one before.

Wear it for a week, and then she'd find me another, she said. I never spoke to my direct manager about this again. She didn't say anything when she saw me with a new N95. She had never said anything when she saw me with the first one, which looked different from the ones the hospital issued.

Many of us felt guilt after a patient loss, guilt that we did not have previously—by which I mean before the pandemic, when we piled into those rooms faster than we could think about it. The worst part was having to call the family and break their hearts with the compound news of the loss after they were unable to visit their loved one. It felt so impersonal to those of us who invest so much in our patients. We started our careers knowing that we could be the last person a patient sees before they die, but never in this magnitude, not with the pressure of their family not being involved in the process. I used to assist patients in doing final care of their deceased loved ones if they wished, so they could perform a last act of love for them.

There were several unexpected deaths of COVID patients, as well as suspicious deaths of friends. I suspected suicides for several people whose cause of death was not disclosed. There had also been an increase in substance overdoses. It seemed that I could not go three weeks without hearing about someone else I knew dying. I heard theories that "they" were hospitalizing minorities to try experimental drugs on them. I was questioned about this by family members and friends. I told them I had not witnessed any such thing. I had a patient who actually worked in a facility where the Tuskegee experiments were conducted. He told me that the records said the patient had syphilis but to not treat. We talked for over 30 minutes. He brought those fears to life in me.

However, I thought about the vaccine trials and how we might not see how it affects people of color due to lack of volunteers. I figured they would end up using the military, which has a higher Black representation. I am a woman of science, but I grew up on home remedies and doctor avoidance because my family was a product of the civil rights era. That White medicine wasn't safe for Black people was just good common sense.

Some of the attention-seeking nurses started working COVID units, taking selfies, and uploading pictures on Instagram. Virtue signaling sucks. But some of them worked there because of the hazard pay, and some because they wanted to help. I was jaded and felt that contracting COVID was inevitable (before I had it, so that turned out to be true). Then I thought about my family and how vulnerable some of my loved ones are. I decided against volunteering to work on that floor, which I regretted when I had a relative land there on a ventilator. I wanted to make sure they had the best chance possible. Luckily, the nurses and doctors on their case were the ones I trusted.

*Trust.* That word was trending when the holiday season started. Health-care workers were asking the community to trust us when we said it wasn't safe: "Don't go to Grandma's; stay home this year so you can still have her in your life next year." Most of the White nurses never imagined sharing real experiences and being dismissed as "fearmongering" or "promoting agendas." They were demoralized when people turned on them as doom-and-gloom party poopers, or even fakes.

However, I was sadly familiar with it. I am a Black woman in Appalachia. Systemic racism has been our trauma for generations. Anyone who hasn't experienced it could believe it was as serious as people thought. Now that the pandemic had thrown everyone into trauma, how could I as a Black person ever explain that we lived at this level of alert most of the time, or that COVID trauma was not the great equalizer White colleagues kept saying it was?

Right after I thought that, the irony hit me that I had not been pulled over by the cops while driving in months, because the only place I went to was to work and my scrubs deterred the officers. My route to work went through a small town where I was, prepandemic, regularly checked out for Driving While Black while running errands.

My coworkers had now lived part of the Black experience for months—by which I mean, they experienced shouting into their community, their country, the world that something was wrong, that we had to work together to save lives, and having people shout back that they were liars. They finally knew how it felt to be that exhausted just trying to do good. They felt the gut-twisting challenge of those little conversations where someone says, "Well, if you don't want to get shot, don't date a drug dealer." I told them to keep speaking up and fight the good fight. We saved lives in that building. Tired people can still save lives.

Next, we had to focus on keeping people out of the building. COVID infections finally truly hit our area that fall. The complaints about sports cancellations disappeared from my timeline. Five health-care facilities had massive outbreaks. People stopped sharing viral posts about not visiting relatives in long-term care. Nine skeptics on my Facebook page were hospitalized, and two were ventilated. A couple of skeptics who did fine gave it to loved ones who did not do well.

Thanksgiving arrived. I knew what would happen. I saw people uploading group pictures, and I cried during the holidays, anticipating what was to come. There were morgue trucks at more of the hospital facilities on my first day back. Three people I knew were in the COVID intensive care unit. My anxiety was at an all-time high.

About the same time that we were trying to pull that spike down, vaccines started rolling. I got mine and shouted from the rooftops to all my Black friends, family, and anyone who would listen. I spoke to Black staff at other hospitals who hesitated, using my nursing clout to tell everyone within the sound of my voice: "Go! Get vaxxed! They're not trying to kill us."

Some did. More did a couple of months later, after I didn't die of it. Then, for a while, the pandemic was in a fuzzy border state. For some it felt over; others denied it ever started, and while infection and death rates were starting to plateau or even fall across the United States, they were rising in other countries. Vaccine access continued to be a critical issue globally; vaccine distrust also continued to be a major issue in Appalachia and other places. Friends and I joked that we hoped someone would sound a buzzer to let us know when the pandemic was officially declared over. And then we adjusted the masks we figured we'd still be wearing this time next year.

Who knew what was to come? But I had a theory: it was going to get worse before it got better, and not just the pandemic. People were edgy, wary, traumatized, and feeling ungracious. During the pandemic, America also began to deal yet again with racial reckoning. I'm not getting my personal hopes up, but I have kids, so maybe I have to hope. Wild pendulum swings are no more a friend to the Black community than performative alliance is. (You know, where someone suddenly realizes how much they need to thank Black nurses, or have Black people on their board of directors, or celebrate Black history month and write about it on social media.) Neither makes substantive changes. Keep fighting the good fight. Exhaustion endures for a night, but the vaccines came. Is equity coming? Maybe. Maybe not. Keep fighting the good fight.

# 13

## Trust Comes Late

WENDY WELCH AND KATHY OSBORNE STILL

*Editor's Note: As the pandemic raged, the nursing shortage proved yet another nationwide crisis. Causes ranged from nurses getting COVID and having to quarantine to quitting outright or leaving specific systems for better pay; in the latter case, nurses often moved to travel companies. Health-care CEOs in some beleaguered states tried to blame the nurses for their decisions to seek more money during a crisis. Of all the lights that COVID shone on disparities of lifestyle, equity, fairness, salary mismatches, and poor working conditions, nursing will endure postpandemic as one of the most previously overlooked and undervalued elements of health-care infrastructure. In order to tell that huge story, this chapter eschews policy and disparity analysis in favor of "a day in the life" storytelling from two nurses who worked COVID units.*

Donna Giles expects to get hit during her emergency room shifts. "It goes with the territory," the 40-year-old registered nurse (RN) said. Giles began working with a large health system a few years before the pandemic began. Patients would arrive at the emergency room doors "having a psychotic episode, or in so much pain they couldn't think straight. They could be violent."

Giles would either handle it or call security, as she deemed necessary. "Even someone tripping will tend to calm down when they see a uniform. Then we clean up the mess, check ourselves for bruises, and go on with our duties." Such episodes rarely even got reported to charge nurses—all in a day's work.

Truth be told, Giles said, she and many of her colleagues found that policies toward nursing violence differed significantly between the official policy manual and actual practice in the hospital. While the health-care system she worked for placed a high value on employee safety at all times in print, if a nurse did report to her supervisor, they would ask, "What could you have done to defuse the situation and keep the patient from turning violent?"

Like so many elements of life, the pandemic changed even these loose parameters.

Malia Watson, a travel nurse and RN with eight years of experience in cardiac care, worked a COVID unit. Giles, also a travel nurse, worked in the intensive care unit (ICU). The two were neighbors by rural standards, overlapped by a couple of years in nursing school, and worked for the same health-care system before deciding to become travel nurses. (Starting pay in the health-care system: $19 per hour; starting pay as a travel nurse: $52 per hour.)

The friends had somewhat different experiences when it came to violence during COVID, as described in this account of that period.

"By the time they get to ICU, the fight is over; they're just literally fighting for their lives; the politics and animosity are gone," Giles said. Patients are often hallucinating, experiencing COVID delirium at this point. "They might think I'm a snake and get combative in that situation, but it's not the same threat as in other situations. Usually at that point we intubate them, put them on a ventilator, and sedate them, so they don't die because they try to rip everything out in their delirium."

Not so Watson's patients, who are still able to speak, lucid, and in a frustrating number of cases will ask for treatments the hospital doesn't give. "Usually it's hydroxychloroquine. They've read something online, they've seen a video, they know what's best for themselves, and they can become violent when told it's not available," Watson said.

Nurses answer per long-standing protocols about any treatment not prescribed by a doctor; they tell the patient that they will let the doctor know about the request. Doctors often navigate the situation by stating the drug is not currently recommended and asking the patient to provide evidence that they need it.

"Doctors can say something to the effect of, 'That is medicine I cannot ethically give you unless supported by evidence,' and then they get to leave the room. The nurses can sometimes take the brunt of patient anger when they try to show their doctor a YouTube video or an American Frontline Doctors article, and it doesn't measure up to evidence." Watson shrugged. "We clean up the mess and try to avoid getting anything broken. And they get better or they get worse. No matter which, they're our patients and we give them everything we've got."

It can be disheartening to know that patients' families have sued hospitals because they felt their nonvaccinated relatives were given substandard care. Such assumption of deviation from full-on best efforts could be considered pure bias, but increasingly it is based on a kind of triage that may or may not be happening, depending on caseloads. Where beds run out, ethical protocols prioritize care for children and those with the best chance of recovery, as deemed by a group of professionals (never one person's decision). This has translated over time and through waves of social media amplification into outright discrimination against the unvaccinated patient.

"Nope," said both Watson and Giles. It doesn't work like that.

First off, nurses have seen hospital staff seek beds across state lines when COVID patients don't have one in their hospital; they know the difference between perceptions of "death panels" and the reality of flying patients in helicopters, allegedly even putting them in private cars according to unconfirmed reports, to reach an available bed someone has spent hours working the phone to hunt down.

More than that, Watson said, "Nursing is a calling. Decisions are made and we're not there. When patients are put in front of us, we give them everything we've got and that's that."

Giles sighed. "It is terrible to lose someone. It's understandable, just like with patient violence, that families will lash out because their loved one didn't make it. They threaten to sue, they take to social media and unload, they say anything in their pain and grief.

But we were there. The last hand a COVID patient holds is a nurse's. We know we did everything possible."

ICU doors were locked because COVID patients couldn't have allowed visitors due to disease spread; this exacerbated conspiracy theories the nurses don't deem worth discussing. Other hospitalized patients were allowed one visitor at a time, or one per day.

"The protocols over time changed, sometimes within a week. But in my ICU, a patient only has a visitor if we know it's almost over," Giles said.

Otherwise the doors stayed locked, the entrance to the hospital staffed by National Guard members tasked with ensuring hospital security. Watson and Giles both have nightmares about family members with guns demanding entrance to their units.

"This is eastern Kentucky we're talking about," Giles said. "Family is everything here. Somebody's going to try it at some point, if they haven't already. It used to be my recurring nightmare when I fell asleep after shifts."

Family members not being in the room is part of what Giles felt contributes to the longevity of bad information leading to bad decisions. A couple of months ago some family members wanted their COVID-ill loved one given a tracheotomy. They had no idea that would have killed her, Giles said, because they hadn't seen her struggle for breath.

"These patients, just rolling over in the bed takes all the life they have. They are gasping for air. It is a terrible thing to see. And of course, no one sees it but us because the families can't be in here. If they do come to ICU, most of the patients have to be sedated to be on ventilators. They don't see that terrible struggle to breathe."

Families are invested in care and trying to make good decisions, the nurses felt, but the deliberate and willful unawareness of some general public members toward what was happening inside COVID wards made everything worse.

"We had the first wave of COVID deaths from nursing homes, but then it was different. We started losing younger patients, and it started getting harder on all of us," said Giles.

Giles and her colleagues filled many body bags during the first 18 months of the pandemic, but something startled her during the summer 2021 viral wave. It didn't register at first, but soon it was hard to ignore, and it shook her.

"They were young." Her voice cracked as Giles offered this succinct summation. Some were just starting careers. Some had children they loved to brag about and share photos of on Facebook. They were in their prime, getting comfortable in life until the COVID-19 virus upended their worlds and devastated their families. They were healthy. They were ready to embrace and subdue the world.

When those deaths started, Giles and colleagues began a mental health rotation system in which nurses covered for each other just so one could take time out for a few minutes and regroup. The increasing amount of young deaths finally started to crack some of the nurses.

"They looked like me," Giles said of the dead. Worse, some looked like her children. She remembers a 19-year-old girl with type 1 diabetes asking, shortly before she died, why the virus was so much harder on her; she thought it killed only the elderly.

Another patient who stands out from the death toll was a 24-year-old man who refused to be put on a ventilator because he thought it would kill him. (He died, after choosing in his last hour of life to be ventilated.) When his mother was notified that her son was going to be incapacitated by a ventilator, she instructed the hospital staff not to vaccinate him while he "couldn't defend himself."

"She wasn't really polite about it," Giles recalled. "Like we were in the business of rendering people helpless and then vaccinating them against their will. All part of the bad info, and who can you trust?"

Do patients conflate the fact that the ventilator is a last resort with how many people die while on ventilators, juxtaposing the cause and the last hope for a cure?

"Yes." Neither Giles nor Watson want to be drawn further on this point, beyond Watson adding, "Bad information is bad information. If five out of six people who go on a ventilator die, must be the ventilator killing 'em. It's that bad out there, the disinformation."

In fact, disinformation is so rampant in the region of the former health-care system these two nurses shared as coworkers that 2022 vaccination rates among nurses in that system hover at an unconfirmed 40 percent. That might be generous. The health-care system isn't talking. Nationwide, a 2021 survey of 4,500 nurses reported 90 percent vaccination rates. The survey is on nursingworld.org.

Giles and Watson are both vaccinated. For the most part, nurses—and other people—who refuse COVID protection confuse and sadden them. "There's like a bewilderment flowing from the vaccinated nurses to the unvaccinated, but the other way, it's more like anger and vitriol. We drank the Kool-Aid; we're flunkies," Watson said with a shrug. This is the main reason that Watson and Giles are pseudonyms; nurses who have spoken to reporters or published pro-vaccine stances on social media have received death threats—Watson included, when she used her real name.

Watson and Giles list the reasons nursing colleagues give for choosing not to vaccinate. Some are straightforward: the vaccine makes you infertile (false); it has side effects not studied, *and* if you as a nurse get any of those side effects, you're going to burn through your sick leave, and insurance isn't going to cover treatment (remarkably specific accusations shared within several large health-care systems nationwide); and the VAERS site.

VAERS stands for Vaccine Adverse Event Reporting System; Giles calls it "Yelp for the health-care world. Anybody can write on that thing; it is literally a big chart of issues people claim to have had after getting a COVID vaccine or booster. My favorite is that two people said getting the COVID vaccine made them retire early. I was kinda hoping for that as my side effect."

Joking aside, the VAERS site has put off several nurses Watson and Giles know. Watson thought part of it had to do with education levels. Licensed practical nurses were, until recently, not required to take microbiology, which she thought would have changed the minds of many vaccine-hesitant colleagues.

Giles disagreed. Minds were made up well before logic and scientific reasoning entered the discussion—if they ever did. She pointed to nurses first saying they wouldn't take the vaccine without FDA approval; when that came, "They said, 'Look what else the FDA approved around here; you gonna trust them?'"

They were referring to OxyContin and the rest of the narcotic painkiller family. Medical mistrust from the fallout of prescription painkillers in communities full of coal miners and loggers, doing physical work and getting addicted to the magic pills prescribed by their trusted family physician, is legendary nationwide. Appalachia is perhaps the American poster child for addiction, and medical mistrust can be considered earned where FDA approval comes into Appalachian perspectives.

The opioid epidemic is not enough to make Watson sympathetic, however. "Yep, we all know how that turned out, and I hope the Sackler family rots in hell. But we still have to fight this pandemic, and our best weapon for that is vaccination."

There is only one vaccine hesitancy that Watson shows sympathy toward, and Giles feels the same. In blunt terms, the more a health-care system insists on vaccination, the more likely their employees might be to evince suspicion, based on the early days of the pandemic.

"What is the first thing everyone is taught about first aid, be it a nurse or somebody taking a CPR class? Assess the scene. You're no good to the electrocuted victim if you get electrocuted too. You gonna drown trying to get someone out of the water? Secure your safety so you are of use to the needy person. That's the first rule of care," Giles started.

Watson picks up the thread. "And it was broken, from day one, for nurses. We didn't get masks, we didn't get PPE, we got told to go in and do our jobs, damn the torpedoes, we were heroes, get in there and be brave. They sent us into battle wearing garbage bags and bandannas. And these are the people who now tell us they've got something to keep us safe, come and get it? Ha! We have no reason to believe them, but we do have reason to believe scientific evidence."

"I don't know anyone who doesn't sympathize with hesitation in trusting the medical profession," Giles said. "I don't know anyone who is just 100 percent always gonna believe and be compliant with what a doctor recommends. Recommendations change, treatment isn't affordable, some things—like having to travel four days a week as a single working mom just to get the prescribed care—that's unrealistic. Treatment gets recommended to patients because it's an across-the-board standard of care and best option, when things should be individualized with case management, so of course that creates barriers to compliance. Our biggest barrier around here used to be access. Now it's suspicion."

"Protocols change; we as nurses know that better than anybody, so maybe because of that someone's hesitant, because what if it changes and you've convinced me to take this thing and later we find out it wasn't safe?" Giles shook her head. "It feels like just another barrier, like I sympathize with someone who doesn't have a car to get to a doctor's appointment and I sympathize with someone who is hesitant because of bad information. Trying to allay that bad info as a nurse doesn't go over well, though. It's a unique challenge.

"Before COVID we would call a case manager, and they'd say, 'Let's make sure we have transport, let's get you home equipment.' This case manager's whole job is 'Let's get you the equipment you need and walk you through to get you the best care we can give despite your personal barriers. We know how to work around those.'

"This is something where we don't know what resources we even have to call. We don't have a case manager to come in and deal with suspicion. In your mind someone else has convinced you I'm the one you can't trust. And I don't find out until we have to intubate you and you say I'm trying to kill you."

For Watson it is a little different, first because she doesn't work in ICU; she has more interaction with coherent, suspicious patients who want to get out of the hospital as fast as possible. Second, Watson is Black, while Giles is White. This gives Watson a leg up on dealing with the medical mistrust patients of color often bring to the hospital along with their overnight bag. Watson is proud that she personally convinced some members of the Black community around her hospital to get vaccinated, largely because she has been available 24/7 to answer their questions, privately and online.

"You don't know tired until you're working a 12-hour shift and spending the next 3 hours convincing someone it's as bad as they say, and then you sit down and do homeschool with your kids," Watson said.

Giles picked up on just how tired nurses were during those days.

"Let's say you've just become a nurse; you're learning some skills, gaining confidence in the job and experience in certain situations. Then let's say a natural disaster happens. So that new nurse says, 'Okay, duty calls; this is what I've been training for,' and they show up at the hospital and dive right in and start helping. And there's such an adrenaline rush. You're ready to run in and save lives, and you say to yourself, 'I'm seeing horrible things but I save lives, this is the moment, this is it, this is what I trained for, my calling and my duty, let's go!'"

"But it will be short, a few hours, a day, a week at the most, running in and saving lives. This is a year and a half and still going. I am so tired. There's no adrenaline rush, just another day of *ugh*. Every day is overwhelming. Full steam ahead for hours in a natural disaster, you run on adrenaline and knowing an end is in sight, every hour makes a difference, you have this one window. Now, they're making us go on and on, and I can tell you for a fact that I have not had adrenaline in a long time, but they're still expecting full steam ahead."

Health-care workers found themselves appreciated by the public at the start of the pandemic, but that changed about the same time younger people began dying. Gone were the days when nurses got a smile and a sincere thank you. Some nurses found themselves verbally attacked in grocery stores or glared at by hate-filled eyes of unmasked people in the checkout lines. It was unsettling, Giles found, "like being permanently gaslit."

Giles and Watson were also attacked by keyboard warriors on social media, people Giles felt would never lash out in person. "They called me a murderer. They said I was killing patients with a ventilator. They gaslight me. They say I'm not giving patients the right treatment. It makes me angry and it makes me defensive."

She became so defensive that "when this peaked about mid-2021, I only left the house to go to work. I was basically on the verge of being locked up in a psych ward. It just got to the point where I couldn't pump my own gas because I couldn't stand to walk into a gas station and see people without masks. All I did was get in my car and go to work and come home."

Her husband packed her lunches and kept the shelf full of Red Bulls for her long shifts at the hospital. He pumped her gas and told her she could quit anytime; he supported whatever decision she made. "I have a great support system," Giles said. "My husband, my family and friends are there for me, and that means so much."

It is part of what pulled her out of the dash from home door to hospital door with nothing else to life. She has started therapy and watches comedy shows when she has time away from her 12-hour ICU shifts. Giles is determined she won't let vicious attacks stop her from a career she enjoys and worked hard to achieve as a lifelong dream, nor will she let the physical or mental drain of the job wear her down.

Watson stayed physically away from her family for a time, fearful of infecting her small children. That might have been the hardest part, knowing her oldest daughter was worried about her, Watson said with a catch to her voice. "When I was home, she would bring me the soap and say, 'Can you smell that, Mom? Okay, you're all right.' But it is about saving lives, and for me it's about being a Black nurse for the Black community, an example and a voice they can trust."

Most of all, she and Giles agree, they aren't going to credit attacks from a public that hasn't seen what they've seen. Giles and Watson grew up in small communities where people cared about neighbors and were eager to help others. The pandemic has revealed another side, and it breaks each of their hearts.

For Giles, it comes back to, "They haven't seen what we've seen. Until you've seen someone die a horrible death, this is too easy to dismiss. There is a big difference between a bad death and a good death. The worst thing that can happen to someone you love is to die scared and alone."

"Let me tell you plainly, and with great sorrow, that these people are not dying peaceful deaths. I don't care how strong or brave anyone is; if you take away their ability to breathe, they panic. We're watching people die horribly, gasping, over and over and over, and

people are just like 'Well, that person's a number.' And they're walking around gas stations with their faces uncovered. People in the
community used to care but now they don't. They don't see the pandemic as a public health matter, let alone a personal thing. They
didn't see how scared they were, didn't see their face."

Giles paused. "That was the worst. These terrible moments of
scared people dying the worst death possible and then we get in the
car and drive home and the rest of the world says this nonverbal
'And?' and goes out to eat and congregates in stores without masks."

Her husband keeps telling Giles she can walk away from work
when she is ready, but that is not in her plans. At this, Watson
laughed. "My husband does not tell me the same. Our kids are little
and we run a farm." Both are determined to stick with nursing and
know they are making a world of difference to patients and families.
Sometimes, they say, that's almost enough.

What do they want to tell the world?

Watson thought for a moment, then said, "I wouldn't trade this
life for anything, but I wish people understood what it's like inside
the hospital walls, and then I wish they'd do all the things that medicine recommends to keep themselves out of them. Like wearing
masks and washing their hands, and getting vaccinated. I don't need
to be called a health-care hero. I need you to get vaccinated so you
don't need a health-care hero. It's our best tool yet."

"I know I'm doing the right thing," Giles said, "but it's so insult-
ing and belittling to health-care workers. The world should see what
we see. They come to my unit to die, and we do everything we can
to save them, but when they die, the unmasked, unvaccinated world
talks about how this isn't any worse than the flu."

She also paused, then said, "If they're lucid, when they know
they're gonna die they reach for us, whether they trusted us before
or not. All that other stuff falls away and it's human connection. In
the end, if we can't save the person in that bed, that's the last act of
care that nurses give. We are the last person to hold their hands,
because we won't let them die alone. Trust comes late, but it comes,
and we're there when it does."

# Part 3

## IMPACT

# 14

## The Two-Sided Pandemic

*Mental Health and Racism before and during COVID-19*

DARLA TIMBO

*Editor's Note: A licensed clinician speaks to mental health concerns predating the coronavirus, caused by being Black in America. It may help contextualize her words to know that two mental health specialists turned down writing this article, on the basis that fear and trauma on the pandemic scale were so new to many White Americans that they could not feel empathy toward Black Americans living daily with the traumatic effects of racism. This chapter focuses on Black experiences with mental health care. Americans are being urged to understand the effects of the pandemic on us as individuals and communities and to seek mental health care when possible; how does this "color-blind" advice affect Black Americans?*

I often sit at my desk after a day of treating clients and stare out the window, thinking about life. So existential, right? Treating a countless number of clients over the years, I've had my fair share of vicarious trauma and distressing situations. My clients suffer from a multitude of mental health issues, ranging from anxiety and depression to racial issues and existing as a Black person in this country. I know, I used the word *existing,* because at times that is what it feels like, just existing! As a Black woman myself, I find it difficult to actually live a fulfilling life in this country without the constant fear that the color of my skin may get me inadequate medical or mental health treatment, because I am not valued. This increased exponentially during the onset of COVID-19. Wow, tough realization for many of us. After sitting, staring out of the window for a few moments, I attempt to take a sigh of relief . . . or do I? I often ask myself, Is there any relief? Is anyone coming to "save" us from the terrifying repercussions of this pandemic—Black people, I mean? I think we may just have to save ourselves.

The years 2020–22 manifested many twists and turns for lots of people. Many of us, including myself, have no idea what the next plot twist will entail. I do know that many of my clients, who are Black, know that the plot will only thicken, as it has for many decades here in America. Not only do Black clinicians and clients deal with the plague of being a member of a marginalized group; we also deal with the plague of racism that comes along with being a part of that group. Black Americans are dealing with a two-sided pandemic, COVID-19 and systemic, deep-rooted racism. This is consistently attacking our proverbial and literal immune systems. Years of fear, mistrust, and stigma have been identified in the literature as significant barriers to Black clients seeking treatment in any sense. This includes medical and mental health treatment. This can be seen in the lesser access to COVID-19-related care Black people have. This has caused continued increase in the underutilization of the available treatment options.[1] These barriers arise from the historic mistreatment of Black people. I find these outcomes to be accurate in my work. Many clients are fearful to be completely vulnerable in treatment due to traumas that they have endured simply because they are Black. I often sit with my lips tight, room filled with silence, while simultaneously screaming inside at the same injustices. Many of my colleagues have identified similar concepts in their practices.[2]

With increasing racial and ethnic diversity in America, it is mandatory that health services be suitable for clients who are seeking these services.[3-5] However, limited information is available that addresses racial and ethnic minority clients' perceptions and satisfaction with the health and psychiatric services they receive during the pandemic of COVID-19.[5,6] It is so apparent in the clients I treat that this two-sided pandemic is not creating any space for a "cure." It is evident that a significant number of doctors and clinicians do not readily consider client diversity, nor do they consider their own cultural competences as being an important part of their ethical conduct.[7] This can be problematic due to ineffective treatment of Black clients. So, why would Black Americans be open to discussing COVID-19 vaccinations and mental health treatment? Would it even be a promising conversation? The answer is fear—fear that even I, as the clinician, experience daily.

The stigma of mental health has shifted for some, but there are still a number of people who are fearful of seeking help within the mental health system. In a given year, about 22 percent of adults in the United States seek mental health treatment.[8] Of those adults seeking mental health treatment, Black clients are much less likely to have access to and receive mental health care than White clients.[9] Compared to other racially diverse groups, Black people are more reluctant to seek mental health treatment for many reasons, including cost, location, lack of services provided, cultural stigma, and mistrust of therapists.[10,11] Some of the arguably more detrimental barriers that deter Black clients include fear of the mental health system, blatant discrimination, and overt/covert racism.[12,13] The ability of Black clients to identify a clinician or doctor with cultural competence could ease apprehension when they are seeking mental health services.[14] So, we need to ask ourselves, Are we making these things accessible to Black people?

### BLACK CLIENTS' RELATIONSHIP TO HEALTH CARE

Relationships have been viewed as an influential part of counseling or medical practices.[15] This research is based on the treatment of White clients and patients over time. Often Black clients and patients are not included in this particular body of research. Because of this, there have been many historical instances that have created disdain toward the field of psychology and medicine. Historically, in the health field, minorities have been misdiagnosed, underdiagnosed, and improperly treated for many concerns.[16-18] Black people have been disproportionately diagnosed and inadequately treated for diagnoses such as psychotic disorders and mood disorders.[18] Many clinicians have characterized Black clients as being oversensitive in the counseling relationship regarding issues of race and also being incapable of meaningful engagement in counseling.[18] This type of characterization and mistreatment has compromised the context for therapy and has accounted for the low utilization rates among Black people and other minorities. Some research articles from the 1950s argued that Black people were not mentally competent enough to even be susceptible to "catching" a mental health diagnosis, and behaviors relative to Black culture have been arbitrated by the dominant culture as pathological and problematic.[12,19,20] For Black people, seeking any type of treatment and remaining engaged once treatment has been initiated will continue to remain difficult if these issues are not addressed.[12]

With this significant fear associated with mental health care, one can only explore the research as it relates to physical health care. Black people are at an increased risk for serious illness if they contract COVID-19 due to higher rates of underlying health conditions (e.g., diabetes, asthma, hypertension, and obesity) when compared to Whites. Black people are more likely to be underinsured or not insured at all, which is an impediment to accessing COVID-19 testing and treatment services. Also, Black people are more likely to work in the service industries that are at risk for loss of income during the pandemic, further reducing access to care. Living in multigenerational households and using public transportation puts them at increased risk for exposure to COVID-19.

FEAR AND MISTRUST

Now that I have shared a bit of literature on the rate at which Blacks are disproportionately treated, let's explore the history that comprises this two-sided pandemic. In the context of mental health settings, the experiences of Black Americans throughout history have shaped the framework of how mental health care is perceived.[12] Twenty-five years after the well-known Tuskegee syphilis study (1932–72) ended, Black Americans continued to fear mental and physical health treatment.[21,22] This study, criticized for not providing informed consent to the men participating in treatment, would be highly unethical by today's standards. Participants were offered free meals and burial expenses, but penicillin was withheld as a treatment option. They were never told they were infected with syphilis as part of the study. This study subsequently tarnished what little trust Black Americans had in doctors and has resulted in substantial fear and underutilization of treatment services, as I discussed previously.[23] While reluctance to engage in mental health treatment was, and still is, a problem for Black clients, it also represented a lack of competence and outreach from the psychological community.

Another instance that was examined by Whaley (2001) looked at negative attitudes toward White mental health clinicians in Black American psychiatric inpatient settings. Both objective and subjective indicators of cultural mistrust indicated that high cultural mistrust scores among Black Americans recently admitted to a psychiatric hospital were associated with more negative attitudes toward White clinicians.[23,24] These findings were consistent with reflection of societal power relationships and cultural values, eliciting cultural mistrust among Blacks. Though Black clients may have exhibited paranoid-like behaviors during interracial therapeutic encounters, it was noted that low self-disclosure, which has been interpreted traditionally as a manifestation of psychopathology, may have been due to cultural mistrust. This behavior indicated a healthy response to a racist society that may be misinterpreted as pathology by mental health professionals, thus causing misdiagnoses and culturally incompetent care.[23-25]

More recent historical events—such as Michael Brown's case in Ferguson, the wrongful arrest of Black Harvard professor Henry Louis Gates, ongoing institutional racism, and the treatment of "illegal aliens" coming to America for a better life—have also created a sense of fear among the culturally diverse, as these events demonstrate the population's general lack of knowledge around multiculturalism and this "pandemic" that many Black people face from birth.

Black Americans' worldviews differ from those of Whites. Concepts such as valuing group relationships over individuality, equality, respect, and cooperation within the community are emphasized in the Afrocentric worldview.[26] Racism affects society as a whole, but greatly affects Black Americans' worldviews.[27] Until worldviews that are ever present in this current pandemic are critically examined, people will remain uneducated regarding the uniqueness of relationships with Black American clients and patients.[28] Continued research, specifically regarding race-based stressors and cultural competence, allows the exploration of various intricacies related to treating Black clients and patients.[3,29] Race-based stressors are thought to have a significant impact on psychological and physical health, so continued research will allow us to examine Black American clients specifically and assess their perceptions of therapy based on a history of oppression, slavery, racism, and mistreatment.[24,30]

The main function of fear is to act as a signal of danger, threat, or conflict, and to trigger the appropriate adaptive responses. Fear arouses defensive behaviors that don't just manifest physically but mentally as well. We learn to fear situations we have been previously exposed to that have caused us pain or distress. This fear subsequently causes us to avoid reencountering these situations, further perpetuating the concept behind this two-sided pandemic.

### RACIAL TRAUMA'S IMPACT ON THE BLACK COMMUNITY

I see three types of trauma emerging from this pandemic. One is interpersonal racial trauma, which occurs within a relationship. This occurs between two people, where race is a factor, and includes bias, discrimination, or violence. One very clear example of this could be interactions with law enforcement officers and the potential outcome. Second, there is also institutional racism that occurs within an organization, including its policies, disciplinary actions, and hiring practices. Lastly, there is systemic racism. This is how organizations and institutions interact and how our political system is structured.

Trauma can affect our mental health, self-esteem, and sense of safety. I've had many experiences where clients have also reported somatic symptoms such as headaches, high blood pressure, gastrointestinal issues, and substance abuse. We already discussed the extensive manifestation of distrust and/or fearfulness causing one to withdraw from social interaction and receiving mental or physical health treatment.

On a larger scale, we do not have access to resources in ways that other racial and cultural groups have, making us less likely to participate in treatment modalities, further perpetuating historical trauma. Dr. Joy Degruy talks about post traumatic slave syndrome being caused by multigenerational abuse.[31] This physical, emotional, psychological, and spiritual abuse has caused significant trauma in the Black community. Many of my clients often speak of "generational curses" that need to be broken. Many of my clients also believe that 2020 and the two-sided pandemic is a continuation of these generational curses. I talk with clients about working through this trauma, but 2020 seems to further engrain the ideals around post traumatic slave syndrome. How can this type of trauma be dismantled?

## ENGAGING BLACK CLIENTS IN TREATMENT AND "SAVING" OURSELVES

I have discussed what this tumultuous year has been like for many Black people. Trying to overcome the historical trauma that has been caused by the medical and psychological world is daunting. As a clinician, I am in the business of helping people to heal. This has been an extremely difficult task this year, and I am sure it will be for many years to come. In an attempt to examine and debunk fear, read on.

When I think about motivation, I think of it as the willingness or desire for us to do something different. We all have a different conceptualization of motivation, in terms of what we are willing to do to achieve success. Having been a part of this historical and generational trauma, I agree it is not easy to engage in meaningful tasks related to treatment. Motivation is one of the most crucial elements in setting and attaining goals and building esteem and courage; it gives us the fortitude to "save" ourselves another day. I've come to the realization that this two-sided pandemic is not helping the situation. I still have some way to go, helping clients dismantle the fear and stigma around mental health treatment and other institutions that have perpetuated this historical trauma for many years, leading up to the beginning of the pandemic.

Just to reiterate, research has indicated that Black Americans have less access to and are less likely to receive mental health or physical health treatments due to multiple barriers encountered in the system, including clinicians' and doctors' overall lack of multicultural competencies, dearth of awareness of cultural issues, bias, and inability to develop real relationships with the therapist.[9] Fear, mistrust, and stigma have all been identified in the literature as some of the most significant barriers to Black people seeking mental health treatment.

Keep in mind, trauma causes anxiety-related symptoms that may manifest in other areas of life. We all experience vicarious trauma- and anxiety-related symptoms through others. Consider the general themes associated with COVID-19 and racism, and the long-term effects, such as generalized anxiety disorder, post-traumatic stress disorder, post traumatic slave syndrome, social anxiety, and phobias. So, I propose conversations around dismantling fear, but even bigger, dismantling systemic and institutional barriers that prevent Black people from trusting these entities. Ways in which Black people can care for themselves are not foreign concepts, but there are concepts that may not have been previously contemplated due to lack of accessibility. Here are some things to consider:

1. Ask yourself, "What do I want to achieve next year? Is this something realistic for me? What do I want to leave behind?"

2. Ask for help from someone you trust. As I discussed, fear is a powerful thing. The statement "If only I . . ." can rear its ugly head, if you let it. Change that statement to "When I . . ." and you will begin taking yourself in the direction you want to go.

3. Ask yourself, "Where do I want to begin?" For example, are you considering counseling or switching doctors? Do your research, learn about the practice and what it provides. These steps will help to empower you.

4. Step out of your comfort zone. Learn about mental health issues that plague the Black community.

5. Set SMART goals: Specific, Measurable, Attainable, Relevant, and Time-Bound. They should be realistic and meaningful—conquering small battles wins the war.

I also encourage us all to gather allies, people who are ready to see and make change, dismantling trauma and bringing racism to its knees.

REFERENCES

1 Cooper-Patrick, L., Gallo, J.J., Powe, N.R., Steinwachs, D.M., Eaton, W.W., Ford, D.E. Mental health service utilization by African Americans and Whites: the Baltimore Epidemiologic Catchment Area follow-up. *Medical Care.* 1999;37:1034–1045.

2 Swanson, M.G., Ward, A.J. Recruiting minorities into clinical trials: toward a participant friendly system. *Journal of National Cancer Institute.* 1995;87:1747–1759.

3 Carter, R.T., Forsyth, J., Mazzula, S., Williams, B. Racial discrimination and race based traumatic stress. In: Carter, R.T., ed. *Handbook of Racial-Cultural Psychology and Counseling: Training and Practice.* New York: Wiley; 2005:447–476.

4 Matthews, A.K., Hughes, T.L. Mental health services use by African American women: exploration of subpopulation differences. *Cultural Diversity and Ethnic Minority Psychology.* 2001;7(1):75–87.

5 Sue, D.W., Sue, D. *Counseling the Culturally Different: Theory and Practice.* New York: Wiley; 1989.

6 Constantine, M.G., Arorah, T.J., Barakett, M.D., Blackmon, S.M., Donnelly, P.C., Edles, P.A. School counselors' universal diverse orientation and aspects of their multicultural counseling. *Professional School Counseling.* 2001;5:13–18.

7 Neighbors, H.W. Mental health. In: Jackson, J.S., ed. *Life in Black America.* Newbury Park: Sage; 1991.

8 National Institute of Mental Health. The numbers count: mental disorders in America. A fact sheet describing the prevalence of mental disorders in America. Washington, DC: NIH; 2013. https://athealth.com/topics/the-numbers-count-mental-health-disorders-in-america/.

9 Mental health: culture, race, and ethnicity. Rockville, MD: Office of the Surgeon General (US); Center for Mental Health Services (US); National Institute of Mental Health (US); August 2001. https://www.ncbi.nlm.nih.gov/books/NBK44251/.

10 Bird, D.C., Lambert, D., Hartley, D., Beeson, P.G., Coburn, A.F. Rural models for integrating primary care and mental health services. *Administration and Policy in Mental Health.* 1998;25:287–308.

11 Fortney, J., Rost, K., Zhang, M., Warren, J. The impact of geographic accessibility on the intensity and quality of depression treatment. *Medical Care.* 1999;37:884–893.

12 Carten, A.J. African Americans and mental health. In: Rosenberg, J., Rosenberg, S., eds. *Community Mental Health: Challenges for the 21st Century.* New York: Routledge; 2006:125–139.

13 Fox, J.C., Blank, M., Rovnyak, V.G., Barnett, R.Y. Barriers to help seeking for mental disorders in a rural impoverished population. *Community Mental Health Journal.* 2001;37:421–436.

14 Patterson, C.H. Multicultural counseling: from diversity to universality. *Journal of Counseling and Development.* 1996;74:227–231.

15 Gelso, C.J., Carter, J.A. The real relationship in counseling and psychotherapy: components, consequences, and theoretical antecedents. *Counseling Psychologist.* 1985;13:155–244.

16 Harley, D.A., Dillard, J.M. *Contemporary Mental Health Issues among African Americans.* Alexandria, VA: American Counseling Association; 2005.

17 Ifetayo, O., McCray, K., Ashby, J., Meyers, J. Use of ifá as a means of addressing mental health concerns among African American clients. *Journal of Counseling and Development.* 2011;89:406–412.

18 Parham, T.A. *Counseling Persons of African Descent: Raising the Bar of Practitioner Competence.* Thousand Oaks, CA: Sage; 2002.

19 Thomas, A., Sillen, S. *Racism and Psychiatry.* New York: Citadel; 1979.

20 Thompson, V.S., Bazile, A., Akbar, M. African Americans' perceptions of psychotherapy and psychotherapists. *Professional Psychology: Research and Practice* 2004;35(1):19–26. doi:10.1037/0735-7028.35.1.19.

21 Lombardo, A., Dorr, G.M. Eugenics, medical education, and the public health service: another perspective on the Tuskegee syphilis experiment. *Bulletin of Medical History* 2006;80:291–316.

22 Washington, H. *Medical Apartheid: The Dark History of Medical Experimentation on Black Americans from Colonial Times to the Present.* New York: Doubleday; 2006.

23 Whaley, A. Cultural mistrust and mental health services for African Americans: a review and meta-analysis. *Counseling Psychologist.* 2001;29(4):513–531.

24 Whaley, A. Cultural mistrust: an important psychological construct for diagnosis and treatment of African Americans. *Professional Psychology: Research and Practice* 2001;32(6):555–562. doi:10.1037//0735-7028.32.6.555.

25 Shelton, D.L. Mistrust of doctors lingers after Tuskegee: many African Americans remain wary—and underserved—a quarter-century after infamous syphilis study. *Washington Post,* April 15, 1997:Z08.

26 Cheatham, H.E. Afrocentricity and career development of African-Americans. *Career Development Quarterly.* 1990;38:334–346.

27 Gillispie, J. F. Construct validation of the multicultural counseling inventory: the contribution of client satisfaction. *Dissertation Abstract International.* UMI No. 9901840, 1999.

28 Katz, J.H., Ivey, A. White awareness: the frontier of racism awareness training. *Personnel and Guidance Journal.* 1977;55:485–489.

29 Clark, R., Anderson, N., Clark, V.R., Williams, D.R. Racism as a stressor for African Americans: a biopsychosocial model. *American Psychologist.* 1999;54:805–816.

30 Pedersen, P. Multiculturalism and the paradigm shift in counseling: controversies and alternative futures. *Canadian Journal of Counseling.* 2001;35(1):15–24.

31 Degruy, J. *Post Traumatic Slave Syndrome.* Joy Degruy Publications, 2017.

# 15

## COVID-19's Enduring Impact on Medical Education

### An Appalachian Case Study

JEFFREY LEBOEUF

*Editor's Note: Building residency programs to train doctors in less populated areas has proven one of the best ways to grow a rural health workforce. The preponderance of residents practice within 50 miles of their residency site after graduation. When the pandemic threatened disruption to graduate medical education, administrators thought fast. Long-term effects could have reduced future medical provision in places that had fought long and hard for respect as learning centers. Such an outcome would have devastating consequences. How could this harm be mitigated?*

The US model of medical education primarily enrolls medical students after completion of an undergraduate degree. The medical school curricula are typically four years, although some have three-year fast-track programs for primary care physicians. The four-year medical school curriculum is bifurcated into two phases: the basic sciences years and the clinical learning years. Following medical school, graduates must complete one to three years of additional postdoctoral training in order to be licensed to practice medicine in any state. To be eligible for board certification in a particular specialty, three to seven years of postdoctoral training are required.

Two accrediting bodies exist for medical schools in the United States. The Liaison Committee on Medical Education (LCME) accredits allopathic medical schools that award the doctor of medicine (MD) degree, while the Commission on Osteopathic College Accreditation (COCA) accredits medical schools offering the doctor of osteopathy (DO) degree. Traditionally, LCME-accredited medical schools are in urban centers and have significant clinical departments at one or more large tertiary teaching hospitals, adjacent to or very near the medical school campus. These schools tend to enjoy state subsidies, and many faculty members are supported by research grants.

Following the two years of basic sciences, third-year medical students most often obtain their clinical training at the university's teaching hospital(s) and clinics. Audition rotations begin in the fourth year; medical students spend time at potential postdoctoral (residency) training sites and other electives.

Osteopathic medical schools are more likely to be in rural or suburban environments. Most osteopathic medical schools do not have a teaching hospital under the same governance; instead they rely on partnerships with community hospitals, physicians, and clinics in larger regional areas for the third and fourth years of training—the clinical years. The medical schools also work with community hospitals and medical staff to create rural residency training programs. This distributive model of education ensures that osteopathic students are fully immersed in community-based medicine and has proven to be a reliable model of producing rural, community-based primary care physicians.

UNDERSTANDING THE CENTRAL APPALACHIAN MEDICAL SCHOOL
AND HEALTH-CARE INFRASTRUCTURE

While the above model holds true across the United States, specifics vary by geographic and cultural elements. As a case study, consider two regional health systems serving central Appalachia and how they intersect with the various medical schools in the same markets.

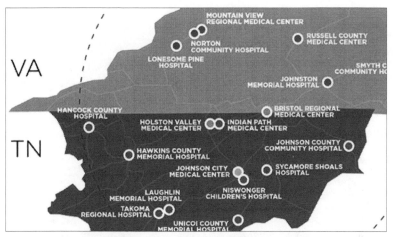

MAP 15.1. Ballad Health hospitals. *Source: Business Journal of Tri-Cities Tennessee / Virginia* and balladhealth.org.

Ballad Health was formed in 2018 via a merger between Mountain States Health Alliance and Wellmont Health Systems. Ballad has hospitals and affiliated clinics in northeastern Tennessee and southwestern Virginia (map 15.1). The organization is operating under a cooperation agreement with the state of Virginia and a Certificate of Public Advantage with the Tennessee Department of Health. As prerequisites to obtaining these agreements, Ballad Health made several commitments to both states, including maintaining existing hospital infrastructure, developing a pediatric trauma center, maintaining costs lower than national averages for patient services, and focusing on population health by investing in health research and graduate medical education, among other things.[1]

Appalachian Regional Healthcare (ARH) operates 13 hospitals in Kentucky and West Virginia (map 15.2), as well as several multispecialty group practices, home health agencies, medical equipment stores, and retail pharmacies. ARH's history traces back to 1956, when it was originally founded by the United Mineworkers of America as the Miners Memorial Hospital Association's (MMHA) facilities. During the early 1960s, MMHA announced a closure of some of the hospitals, so Appalachian Regional Hospitals formed

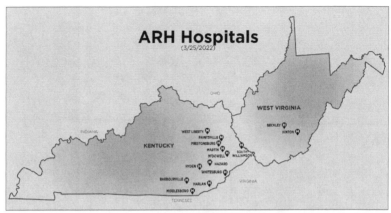

MAP 15.2. Appalachian Regional Healthcare hospitals. *Source:* Appalachian Regional Healthcare, https://www.arh.org/about_us.aspx.

and purchased the MMHA hospitals. In 1986, the name was changed to Appalachian Regional Healthcare.[2]

Also serving the central Appalachian region are four osteopathic medical schools and four allopathic medical schools. Osteopathic schools are located in Harrogate, Tennessee; Blacksburg, Virginia; Pikeville, Kentucky; and Lewisburg, West Virginia. Allopathic schools are located in Lexington, Kentucky, and in Roanoke, Virginia, as well as Knoxville and Johnson City, both in Tennessee. While these schools are on the periphery of the Ballad and ARH service areas, they are included in this analysis since Ballad and ARH provide clinical training opportunities to allied health, nursing, and medical students from the medical schools, nursing schools, and allied health programs located in those communities.

COMMUNITY HOSPITAL AND AFFILIATED CLINICAL
INTERSECTIONALITY IN MEDICAL EDUCATION

Local community health systems and affiliated clinics enjoy a mutually beneficial relationship with institutions of higher learning in the region. Communities depend on local colleges and universities to be workforce-development incubators for the growing health-care needs of the population. Health care is a unique system in many

ways, including but not limited to the diversity of educational requirements and specialization of professionals required to deliver
care. Many health-care careers include clinical rotations or on-site
field experiences as key components of their curricula. For this reason, hospitals and clinics will often have nursing, physical therapy,
radiation technology, occupational therapy, physician assistant, and
medical students enrolled in field experiences under the supervi-
sion of volunteer adjunct faculty who are practicing professionals
in these disciplines. Some rural training sites become overly saturated with learners and have a limited number of volunteer faculty
members. Clinical adjunct faculty members often express feelings of
being overburdened with teaching, evaluating, and managing students, as well as their medical practice responsibilities.

EARLY COVID IMPACT ON MEDICAL EDUCATION AND THE RESPONSE

As Americans became cognizant of the potential danger of the
emerging SARS-CoV-2 (COVID-19) pandemic, both health systems discussed here began meeting within themselves to plan responses and to evaluate the impact of various population-exposure
scenarios.

Each system vowed to ensure that all decisions were clinically
based (in other words, for the good of the patients). Both identified several immediate issues: a shortage of personal protective
equipment (PPE); fear for the safety of learners; a need to preserve
financial resources and key health-care supplies; and an inability
to rapidly test students and workers. ARH removed many nonvital
personnel, including students, from clinical environments. Some
respiratory therapy programs and certified registered nurse anesthetists (CRNA) training programs fast-tracked the graduation of
their students in their final year of training in order to respond to
the pandemic at ARH facilities. Some nursing students who were
already performing key functioning roles continued to provide vital
nursing care. This included staffing intensive care units (ICUs). Like
ARH, Ballad kept CRNA students in place, due to their ability to
provide intubation and ICU management.

Physician assistant student rotations and medical student rotations were suspended, as Ballad and ARH each sought to remove nonvital personnel from harm's way and preserve personal protective equipment. Each system also discontinued most clinical training of nursing students, respiratory therapy students, and other allied health students, except as previously described. Many medical schools quickly designed distance learning (i.e., online rotations) to ensure that medical students remained on cycle through the end of the academic year, June 30, 2020. Most medical schools were well versed in using distance learning technologies, such as Microsoft Teams, Blackboard, Zoom Video Communications, and Cisco Webex, to name a few, and quickly adapted to at-home distance learning for both preclinical sciences students (first and second year), as well as students on clinical rotations.

Rural health-care systems suffered a devastating effect from the national shutdown in March and April 2020. Although COVID-19 caseloads were relatively low, hospitals and clinics took a severe economic blow due to the delay of elective procedures and surgeries, as well as routine office visits and laboratory and radiological tests. Inpatient and outpatient clinical volume plummeted to below 30 percent of pre-COVID levels. Both health systems had to furlough 8 to 10 percent of employees.[3,4] Most community providers (nonsystem health-care providers) were also adversely impacted financially.

Pre-COVID, telehealth was used sporadically in a few disciplines, radiology being a prime example; telehealth also connected rural health-care teams to urban centers of excellence for subspecialty consultations. ARH, for example, has telemetry connectivity from each of its ICU units to a central hub for real-time subspecialty monitoring and communications. During COVID, telehealth became the dominant way primary care physicians maintained periodic office visits and wellness checks with patients. Schools began to ensure that students were being trained to navigate a telehealth visit.

By the beginning of the new academic year on July 1, 2020, most medical schools and clinical core sites had enough retrospective data on PPE surplus and use rates to comfortably reopen student clinical training. Some medical schools and regional nonprofits assisted with PPE procurement.

Both US medical licensing exams, the US Medical Licensing Examination (USMLE) and the COMLEX-USA, administered by the National Board of Osteopathic Medical Education (NBOME), are taken in three parts during the course of one's medical education. The first level must be passed before a medical student can begin their third year of medical school. The second step has two components: a cognitive evaluation and a performance evaluation. Both must be completed before graduating medical school. The final part, Level 3, must be taken after one year of postdoctoral (residency) training. COMLEX-USA's Level 2 Performance Evaluation (PE) and the USMLE's Step-2 Clinical Skills (CS) each require a hands-on patient-focused exam in a simulation center clinical testing laboratory. Both NBOME and COMLEX suspended this exam in response to COVID-19 (it was permanently canceled later). For the students caught in this coronavirus limbo, it was unclear when or how they could take this USMLE Step-2-CS or the COMLEX Level-2-PE in their training. This caused significant anxiety among medical students.[5,6]

In normal times, much of the medical school fourth year is used to explore residency programs by going on two- or four-week audition rotations. During the COVID-19 pandemic, most of these audition rotations were suspended. Day-long formal interviews and hospital tours were likewise suspended and replaced with virtual interviews using web-based meeting software. Thus, fourth-year medical students were forced to navigate the audition and application processes for matching into a residency program much differently during the pandemic. Because students did not incur the travel expenses to get to the formal interviews, many opted to apply to many more—in most cases, dozens—of residency programs. Residency program directors and selection committees were deluged with several times more than the normal numbers of applications. For the most part, they did not meet the candidates in advance, neither via audition rotations nor formal on-site interviews, compounding the difficulties of selection.

LONG-TERM IMPACTS OF COVID-19 ON WORKFORCE DEVELOPMENT

Health system leaders predict several lasting impacts on clinical education post-COVID. Each rotation, or clinical learning experience, will be analyzed to see how much of it must be at the bedside or in the clinic, versus how much can be virtual. Pure virtual rotations may remain in those disciplines that lend themselves more toward telehealth (radiology and psychiatry, for example, as well as some electives). Didactics, group study sessions for board exams, and clinical case reviews may largely remain virtual. In-person rotations will be more focused on diagnosis and management skills. Students and faculty making rounds on inpatients will be in much smaller groups to minimize nosocomial infections (that is, infections acquired in hospitals).

The orientation, or "onboarding," of student learners at hospitals and clinical sites will focus more on infection control procedures, proper use of personal protective equipment, contact tracing, and other lessons learned from this pandemic. Part of orientation will include initial monitoring/screening and daily monitoring for two weeks. New technologies are also being evaluated, such as temperature-taking stations and radio-frequency identification badges to monitor handwashing. The COVID-19 vaccine will be added to the prerequisite boosters and screenings.

Telehealth rotations may be needed to educate students on how to teach their patients to self-obtain key diagnostic variables, such as temperature checks, blood pressure readings, and glucose levels. Telehealth will remain the preferred way to conduct periodic wellness checks for medication management of patients with well-managed chronic conditions. These visits are safer for most patients, since the risk of acquiring clinic-borne infections, such as influenza, from other acutely sick patients is eliminated. How will the healthcare system ensure that these patients have reliable internet service, web cameras, and an ability to navigate the telehealth portal? How can systems support reliable at-home diagnostic equipment and knowledge of their correct use to ensure that providers are making sound care plans based upon reliable clinical data?

During the 2020–21 residency match cycle, ARH and Ballad Health joined most health systems throughout the nation in suspending all in-person audition rotations for medical students (those two-week- or four-week-long rotations at residency program sites) so students and program faculty could assess the goodness of fit for ongoing training. Ballad and ARH have moved to virtual interviews with qualified applicants. The decision to resume in-person audition rotations was based on the desire to give the programs and the candidates as accurate a picture as possible. The virtual interviews were noted to be challenging due to technical and other reasons; it will be interesting to follow the performance of the class of 2021 in comparison to other classes that benefited from audition rotations and in-person interview days. Several national associations and accreditation councils are wrestling with the issue of promulgating future guidelines regarding audition rotations.

Ballad Health and ARH anticipate training roughly the same numbers of learners as pre-COVID; however, each rotation will have to be individually analyzed for content and learning modalities.[7,8] It is important to note, finally, that the number of people applying to osteopathic medical school as the pandemic draws (hopefully) to a close has increased 18 percent.[9] Allopathic medical schools across the country are also reporting the same 18 percent increase in applications.[10] Medical schools, of both traditions, are applying to their accrediting bodies for new campuses and class-size increases.

Each year a few new medical schools form. These expansions involve processes that take considerable investments of time, financial resources, and curricula development. The United States may soon face a bottleneck, as health systems like ARH and Ballad become overly saturated with learners and cannot take the expanded class sizes. Since the Balance Budget Act of 1997 created caps on graduate medical education, hospitals with existing residency and fellowship programs receive no additional reimbursement from the Centers for Medicare and Medicaid Services (CMS) for expanding their training programs.[11] Perhaps the nation will seek to solve the geographic misdistribution of its physician workforce through public policy changes. How legislators and federal health regulators and policy makers choose to incentivize health systems to create rural primary care residency programs matters. Similarly, the nation's policies, health care, and educational systems should ensure that students willing to train for practice as rural primary care physicians have the means and support to do so.

REFERENCES

1 COPA & Cooperative Agreement. Ballad Health merger. https://www.balladhealth.org/copa. Accessed June 13, 2022.
2 Appalachian Regional Healthcare (ARH). https://www.arh.org/about-us/. Accessed June 13, 2022.
3 Paavola, A. Appalachian Regional Healthcare furloughs 500 employees. Becker's Hospital Review, March 27, 2020. https://www.beckershospitalreview.com/finance/appalachian-regional-healthcare-furloughs-500-employees.html.
4 Paavola, A. Ballad Health to furlough 1,300, expects cash flow drop of $150M. Becker's Hospital Review, April 8, 2020. https://www.beckershospitalreview.com/finance/ballad-health-to-furlough-1-300-expects-cash-flow-drop-of-150m.html.
5 COMLEX-USA Level 2-PE. NBOME. https://www.nbome.org/assessments/comlex-usa/comlex-usa-level-2-pe/. Accessed June 13, 2022.
6 USMLE Suspending Step 2 Clinical Skills Examination. Coronavirus Research Center. https://COVID.usmle.org/announcements/usmle-suspending-step-2-clinical-skills-examination. Accessed December 8, 2020.
7 Maria Braman, MD, chief medical officer, Appalachian Regional Healthcare, interview with author, May 27, 2020.
8 Matthew Loos, MD, chief academic officer, Ballad Health, interview with author, May 27, 2020.
9 Raymond, R. "The Fauci effect": applications are up 18% at osteopathic medical schools. The DO, December 2, 2020. http://thedo.osteopathic.org/2020/12/the-fauci-effect-applications-are-up-18-at-osteopathic-medical-schools/.
10 Budryk, Z. Medical schools call 18 percent increase in applications "Fauci effect." The Hill, December 7, 2020. https://thehill.com/policy/healthcare/529045-medical-schools-call-18-percent-increase-in-applications-fauci-effect.
11 Davis, P.H. The effects of the Balanced Budget Act of 1997 on graduate medical education. Council on Graduate Medical Education Resource Paper, March 2000. https://www.hrsa.gov/sites/default/files/hrsa/advisory-committees/graduate-medical-edu/resource-papers/March-2000-balanced-budget.pdf. Accessed June 13, 2022.

# 16

## COVID-19 and Type 2 Diabetes

*A Seesaw of Reckoning*

BRITTANY LANDORE

One of the most prevalent chronic illnesses in Appalachia, rural or urban, is diabetes mellitus type 2. Patients with diabetes struggle to maintain control over their blood sugar levels and also to defend themselves from other illnesses because they are immunocompromised. COVID-19 has taken advantage of the diabetic patient's compromised position and made it one of the most common predisposing conditions for COVID-19.

I work in a health-care system that runs more than 20 rural clinics and a few hospitals. Because so many people in my Appalachian hometown suffer from diabetes, I interviewed several physicians about treating diabetic patients during the pandemic. Part of the discussion includes figuring out what that treatment was and why it presented unique challenges to treat diabetic patients who developed COVID-19.

STEREOTYPES VERSUS REALITIES

The Appalachian region has long been publicized in the media as overrun with uneducated working-class citizens. This is a stereotype we like to reject. Besides, nobody had a good handle on how to educate the public on COVID-19 when it started, so we were all ignorant together. It didn't help that mixed messages about how to stay safe went rippling across America because of clashes between scientific institutions and politicians. So it wasn't just Appalachians who were poorly educated about the COVID-19 signs and symptoms, but the fact that so many people in the region were unsure or unaware caused many to wait until their symptoms were severe before seeking treatment.

Providers struggled, prepandemic, to make diabetic patients understand that they were immunocompromised overall. So it is only to be expected that, as the pandemic raged, diabetic patients did not always take the appropriate extra measures befitting their health status to prevent illness from COVID-19. Diabetic patients in my clinic said they continued to travel, go shopping, or go on vacations to crowded beaches; many of these conversations were held after the patient had contracted COVID-19.

According to the CDC, people of any age who have been diagnosed with chronic kidney disease, chronic obstructive pulmonary disease, an immunocompromised state from a solid organ transplant, obesity (a body mass index of 30 or more), serious heart conditions (heart failure, coronary artery disease, cardiomyopathies), sickle-cell disease, or type 2 diabetes mellitus are at increased risk of severe illness from COVID-19.[1] In the early stages of the pandemic, COVID-19 was widely publicized as a disease that mainly affected the respiratory system, so naturally, people in the general population with preexisting pulmonary conditions were more concerned than most about contracting the virus. We have a lot of black lung patients in our service area and have held many conversations with them to reassure, assess, and advise.

However, it has become apparent that some of the sickest patients in our rural region had diabetes mellitus without any preexisting pulmonary conditions. One diabetic woman I spoke to stated that she didn't believe she was at risk for COVID because her lungs were healthy and she had never smoked. She didn't understand that diabetes is a serious illness causing complications that placed her in the high-risk community to contract COVID-19. Many people, both patients and acquaintances outside the clinic, had this same mindset; they went about their day-to-day life, vacationing in summer and gathering with family over the winter holidays, without taking extra precautions to guard their compromised health.

### APPALACHIAN PHYSICIAN EXPERIENCES

I spoke with several senior physicians in my health-care system about their experiences to see if the attitudes they found in their patients matched those of my own patients. To preserve privacy, all names have been abbreviated to an initial.

Dr. C cared for a hospitalized COVID-19 patient who had contracted the virus while on family vacation to her favorite seaside town. This patient joined others who soon discovered that, though they felt safe staying outside and enjoying sun-filled vacation days on the beach, they were inadvertently bringing a deadly virus home with them and spreading it to those who had tried to stay safe by not leaving their hometown.

Dr. C joined other doctors in noticing what appears to be a cycle of illness among COVID-19 patients in rural Appalachia. Dr. M said patients would come to the hospital with a positive test and mild cough, improve after a couple of days, and be sent home and advised to return to the hospital if their symptoms became more severe. The patient would then come back to the hospital three or four days later and would require supplemental oxygen. On the fifth day, the now-hospitalized patient's cough and shortness of breath would become worse and they would need higher amounts of supplemental oxygen. By the eighth day of illness, patients would develop what is called a cytokine storm, a release of inflammation molecules that can cause damage to cells. Between days ten and fourteen, the patient would form a microembolism.

A microembolism is a very small blood clot that forms in small blood vessels. Over time, these tiny blood clots move through the vessels, sticking together with other small blood clots; if you're thinking of rolling a snowman, the concept is similar. Eventually these microembolisms become large enough to stop the blood flow through larger blood vessels. When the blood flow stops to the heart, a myocardial infarction (heart attack) can develop; when blood flow stops to the brain, the patient could have a stroke. When blood flow stops to kidneys, they can no longer filter toxins.

The human body produces urine in order to get rid of excess fluid, excess electrolytes (like sodium, potassium, and calcium), and waste products from metabolism. If there is too much extra fluid in the body, swelling of the extremities and other organs can develop. If there are too many electrolytes in the body, it can affect one's heart rate, the function of organ systems, and muscle function; it can also cause brain swelling. Waste products of metabolism not released from the body harm brain and liver function, as well as produce gout.

Damage that is caused from lack of blood flow to the heart, brain, lungs, kidney, or any other major organ system can lead to permanent deficits in the function of that organ. The microemboli in the diabetic COVID-19 patients would often spread to many locations and cause multiple organ failure. Doctors would carry out what was referred to as therapeutic anticoagulation (using medication to thin the blood) to try and manage small blood clot production. But some providers found that after patients initially improved and were sent home, they would later develop aneurysms (swelling of a large blood vessel that leads to the portion of the vessel wall bursting), which led to their unfortunate demise.

From speaking with Dr. P, the most common treatment plan for COVID-19 patients while in the hospital originally consisted of a medication called Plaquenil (brand name for hydrochloroquinine): 400 mg twice daily for one day followed by 200 mg daily for five days. Dr. P noticed no direct negative side effects of the medication on kidney function in diabetics from Plaquenil, but his main concern was their dehydration status. In replenishing diabetic patient fluids, providers had to make sure they inadvertently didn't cause an acute kidney injury by giving too much fluid, too fast, through an IV (similar to a balloon bursting). An acute kidney injury leaves the kidney with difficulties in producing urine, as well as getting rid of waste products that are normally cleared by these body cleaning machines.

The original treatment plan in spring 2020 involving Plaquenil called for high doses of fluids; for diabetic patients, providers would be extra cautious by carefully monitoring creatinine clearance. Creatinine is a protein that is filtered through the kidneys easily; by measuring how much creatinine has been filtered out of the blood into the urine, providers can measure how well the kidney is functioning. Over time, the treatment course recommendations changed. By autumn we were using a medication called remdesivir and steroids like dexamethasone for ten days, after a study called the RECOVERY Trial. Dr. F spoke to me about how he followed the RECOVERY Trial to develop his treatment plans. According to Dr. F's recollection, patients needed to meet certain qualifications to be started on treatment with remdesivir, including requiring 2–6 L supplemental oxygen first. (As a resident, I wasn't allowed to give this treatment.) Another colleague discussed how new studies had shown that Plaquenil has the potential to be harmful to COVID-19 patients. An unfortunate side effect of steroid medication is elevated blood glucose. When blood glucose levels become too high, this can lead to kidney damage, nerve damage, and at dangerously elevated levels it can even cause diabetics to go into a coma. Over and over again, I wish we could have explained to diabetic patients how difficult it would be to treat them if they became severely ill with COVID. Good options for other patients were not for them.

Most providers I talked with started their hospitalized diabetic COVID patients on sliding-scale insulin even if they didn't take insulin normally at home. Placing all diabetics on insulin when they were admitted to the hospital allowed providers to maximize blood sugar control prior to starting treatment with steroids like dexamethasone.

Dr. R had several patients who actually required continuous insulin administration through an IV drip while in the hospital, because their blood glucose headed into the 500s range after treatment by steroids. (A normal blood sugar is below 100.) A colleague discussed how it's more difficult to maintain blood glucose control in diabetics during hospital stays for many reasons. Controlling blood glucose in the hospital setting can be tricky, when patients are being fed food that they may not normally eat; sometimes patients are able to control their blood sugar at home much better with their own diet than with what is provided by the cafeteria's diabetic menu.

Another reason is because these patients are sick before they get sick, which sounds odd, but illness will commonly increase blood sugar levels as a by-product of the body naturally trying to fight off infection. Limited activity while in the hospital also makes it hard to control diabetic blood sugar. Patients are often able to help manage their blood sugar at home with exercise, while in the hospital with COVID-19, patients are quarantined to their hospital room, often even bedbound due to their requirement for breathing assistance devices.

Dr. X cared for COVID-positive diabetic patients in a clinic; he treated patients' initial symptoms of aching joints and fever with ibuprofen and advised them to immediately start treatment with 81 mg aspirin. He was hopeful that early administration of aspirin would prevent microembolisms. He also treated all COVID-19 diabetic patients who did not require hospitalization with Plaquenil, azithromycin, and dexamethasone by mouth. Diabetic COVID-19 patients were also advised to immediately purchase a pulse oximeter machine to periodically monitor their oxygen levels, even if they didn't have any underlying lung disorders. Dr. X recommended his patients go to the hospital if their oxygen levels dropped below 94 percent. Good outcomes resulted when patients followed this treatment regimen, and to the best of Dr. X's knowledge, his at-home patients did not suffer from microembolism as an additional complication of COVID-19 infection.

### DIABETIC LIFE AFTER DIAGNOSIS OF COVID-19

After patients are discharged from the hospital, normally hospitalist providers are not privy to their patient's follow-up care. Unfortunately, COVID-19 has not changed that lack of follow-up information shared with the hospitalist providers. It can be difficult to keep the lines of communication open between outpatient physicians and hospitalist services in rural areas at the best of times; in a health crisis that stretched working hours and existing systems to the breaking point, this follow-up repeatedly fell by the wayside. Often times, COVID-19 diabetic patients were discharged to a rehabilitation facility with supplemental oxygen. Unless the patient had an unfortunate degradation in their condition requiring rehospitalization, hospitalists too often had no way of knowing how their patients were progressing—although one doctor shared with me that she found out in a touching way. One of her patients returned to the hospital after discharge and brought Dr. P and the hospital team a meal in gratitude for their efforts to care for her.

Physicians and health-care professionals have made wonderful progress in treating COVID-19 by sharing information across the country, but the range of additional health problems many patients may face in the future is still unknown. Continued loss of taste, joint aches, headaches, and fatigue are emerging as "long hauler" symptoms, but as with COVID itself, they are puzzling in their behavior. They affect different patients, with different symptoms; there are no patterns yet.

This uncertainty is especially true for diabetic COVID patients. Will they have immunity from the virus reinfecting them after testing positive for COVID-19? How many diabetics participated in the clinical trials for the Moderna and Pfizer vaccines? One provider had already taken care of patients who were reinfected with the virus roughly a month after their previous infection. Another had concerns about the patients developing new issues after COVID treatment: brain fog, forgetfulness, and anxiety are growing in public awareness, but the list is larger.

Some patients seemed to have difficulty tolerating the treatment of high-flow oxygen while in the hospital and would often try to take off their supportive oxygen devices, stating they couldn't stand it any longer. Some providers voiced concerns that some of the patients may possibly be at risk for developing post-traumatic stress disorder after COVID-19 infection treatment. Another doctor was more concerned about heart problems that had occurred during COVID-19 infection, noting that many diabetic patients were developing cardiomyopathy. Cardiomyopathy impairs the heart's ability to pump blood to the rest of the body. As mentioned before, patients may suffer from chronic organ failure issues for the remainder of their lives after microembolism development as a poor outcome of COVID-19 infection.

Though treatment plans for COVID-19 have been developed, not every patient recovers in the same way. A colleague suggested it's an all-too-easy mistake to become overconfident while treating COVID patients; just about the time one believes something will work for a diabetic patient each time, it doesn't on the next person. Patients are individuals. Providers have done the best we can to anticipate poor outcomes; unfortunately, poor outcomes come in all shapes and sizes.

One provider said it was difficult to parse all the misinformation that was being shared in an attempt to develop a treatment plan. Sifting through research was like riding a seesaw; a technique would be up one week, down the next. It also seemed to be an issue that providers weren't collecting adequate samples for COVID-19 testing; patients were initially testing negative and then when retested showed positive results. This was in part due to how well the swabs captured specimens from the patient.

Even though unique problems were likely with each patient, over time COVID-19 has shown an overall pattern to disease progression that we now work hard to preemptively treat during every step in that progress. Most of the physicians felt more comfortable after a year of treating COVID diabetic patients than they did initially, but still felt it's imperative to keep up to date with what research is showing to be effective in COVID treatment currently. The information changes fast. The seesaw is also on steroids.

It appeared to be a consensus among health professionals in rural areas that until a vaccine was created for COVID-19, this virus would reign as the number-one health concern across the globe. This is somewhat ironic in an area beset by so many other crises: diabetes, substance use disorder, chronic obstructive pulmonary disease, and black lung, to name a few. These haven't gone away, and there is no vaccine for most of what we would have called our major crises before the pandemic. As physicians, we still face those challenges.

CDC GUIDANCE FOR DIABETIC PATIENTS

Still, even as vaccines protect us, COVID-19 remains at the forefront of our patient care, and we will continue to urge patients (diabetic and nondiabetic) to follow CDC guidelines for avoiding infection, limiting spread, and getting vaccinated. Unfortunately, most of the physicians I spoke with said many of their diabetic COVID patients were uneducated and honestly didn't know what to do to prevent illness initially. They also had lower incomes, unable to stock up and stay home. They seemed unaware that, according to the CDC, the best way to protect yourself and reduce the risk of spreading COVID-19 was to limit interactions with other people as much as possible.

The CDC also recommended certain precautions, now well known to everyone, to prevent contracting COVID-19. Recommendations included washing your hands often with soap and water for at least 20 seconds, wearing a mask, and social distancing. Unfortunately, patients were not following recommendations as hoped. Monitoring their health daily was the one thing diabetic patients tended to do already, but not because of CDC guidelines; it had become a lifestyle (for some, not all) due to their type 2 diagnosis.

The early CDC list of common signs and symptoms of COVID-19 included shortness of breath, cough, and fever. However, the way the disease assailed patients was not always via the signs they were looking for, if they were aware of the CDC list at all. Some patients developed more gastrointestinal symptoms like nausea, vomiting, and diarrhea. Also, by autumn 2020, providers reported feeling that the symptom lists couldn't be trusted anymore, as patient experiences varied so widely. Some patients reported just feeling tired and running a mild fever initially before testing positive for COVID-19. Other patients required high-flow oxygen to maintain a safe oxygen level but felt absolutely fine and denied having any symptoms of illness. The seesaw of symptoms moved as fast as the seesaw of treatment suggestions. By the time Thanksgiving and Christmas brought spikes in infection as people ignored guidelines and gathered in nonhousehold groups, most bets were off on presenting symptoms that suggested COVID.

WERE WE READY IN RURAL APPALACHIA FOR COVID-19?

As the disease spread across the nation, people everywhere, including our rural area, seemed to become more aware of recommendations for prevention and yet also polarized: either aware and compliant, or openly defiant (still aware, just unwilling). Even as the holiday spike arrived, one physician commented that at the same time, thanks to the local media and numerous national television and radio commercials, awareness of COVID-19 household best practice procedures had saturated the region. That said, many physicians still believed that patients did not fully understand how widespread the virus was in our part of rural Appalachia. Accustomed to being passed by in all things city-esque, they still thought of New York and Los Angeles as hot spots, not our little towns—but we had two spikes, the first rising slowly in October then jumping at Thanksgiving and running right through the holidays. The spike in March 2021, as vaccine rollouts combined with COVID fatigue, sent people out to shops, restaurants, and churches without masks or social distancing. The fact that the virus took until October to reach us in significant numbers added to some people's belief that we were safe in our corner of the world.

Some local physicians believed their facilities were well equipped for the crisis at hand, having benefited from the additional six months it took for the virus to reach us from metropolitan cities to rural communities. As soon as the "newer" medication treatment remdesivir was available on the market, Dr. W reported, he was contacted by a distributor to determine whether any patients at his facility were candidates for the treatment. When it turned out one of Dr. W's patients was eligible, it was available within 24 hours.

Most of the providers I spoke with felt that area hospitals could have done more to be prepared. After all, they had six months during which rural cases rose slower than the rest of the nation. During that additional time, emails and online information were flying between doctors in various areas talking about what they were trying and how well it was working. Area hospitals could have done more to be prepared.

Several providers felt that the hospitals could have stocked up better on masks, gowns, and gloves so that special precautions to conserve used personal protective equipment (PPE) didn't have to be utilized. Other providers thought in the extra time Appalachia had to prepare, they could have established better protocols to limit staff exposure by more efficiently scheduling specific nurses and physicians to see only COVID-positive patients daily. That would limit possible cross-contamination in the hospital setting. It was also suggested by one provider that the hospitals could have better prepared the COVID-designated centers in the hospital so that there was more space to care for COVID-positive patients with more hospital bed availability and to ensure that there was only one COVID-positive patient per hospital room.

A few providers stated that their facility never ran out of PPE, and there were even policies set in motion to reprocess masks so they could be reused if resources became scarce. Most felt that facilities as of Thanksgiving 2020 were never overrun with COVID-19 patients. They always had available beds in negative pressure rooms (specialized hospital rooms that have their own ventilation system so diseases that are spread through the air don't get dispersed throughout the hospital's ventilation system) where additional COVID-positive patients could be treated if necessary. In both waves mentioned, the supplies, personnel, and beds held; we all worked hard to try to prevent another wave by encouraging vaccinations. When it did come, we felt even more ready.

Though all the physicians I spoke to working in rural Appalachia couldn't agree about their facility's level of preparedness for the COVID-19 pandemic, they could agree on the level of support they felt from coworkers. All the physicians I talked to said without exception that they were scared, but they didn't feel alone. They appreciated how so many workers throughout their care systems were able to come together to take care of the community. Janitors cleaned with the knowledge that lives depended on it. Nurses worked double shifts. Respiratory therapists were everywhere, doing everything they could. Everyone knew it was all for one, or all went down together.

Dr. L mentioned the great peace of mind she had, knowing that her coworkers were doing everything possible to keep not only themselves protected but coworkers and other patients in the hospital as well. One hospital used extra-long IV lines and kept IV pumps outside of the patient's room with the doors shut to help reduce risk of exposure. Another doctor worked in a small hospital that didn't have a pulmonologist regularly; during the height of the pandemic's first wave, two pulmonologists were brought in on alternate weeks to provide continual care so that the community had coverage 24 hours a day, seven days a week. One physician stated her facility also instituted a willing participant prayer at the beginning and end of each work shift. "God was with us," this provider proudly exclaimed.

After speaking to multiple doctors who have been integral to the care of patients in rural Appalachian communities, it appears that the emergence of the COVID-19 pandemic became a "leveler in the medical community," as described by Dr. L, who went on to explain it has been a brand-new problem for physicians who just completed their training, as well as providers who have been working for the past 30 years; we are all students of this virus, no matter how many years we have been practicing.

Due to this virus being a new and unique issue for providers to manage, we had to develop unique ways to provide patient care. Doctors stepped in to do some of the regular nursing duties—such as managing the IV pumps and providing insulin administration while completing patient visits. In part, this was to try and conserve PPE as much as possible and in part compensating for the low number of workers in the hospitals during the crisis. Everyone was trying to make sure patient care was not limited, even though there was a limit to personnel on hand.

One physician commented that he felt, during the height of the COVID crisis in his community hospital, that everyone worked together as a team much better than usual. I can say from experience that we all pitch in where needed. Crises sometimes bring out the best in a team with common goals—keeping as many people alive as possible, including ourselves.

A FEW SUGGESTIONS FOR DIABETICS

According to the American Diabetes Association (ADA), the risk of a diabetic mellitus patient getting very sick from COVID-19 is likely to be lower if their diabetes is managed well.[2] The ADA further explains that when diabetics have fluctuating blood sugars, they are generally at a risk for a number of diabetes-related complications. Heart disease and other complications in addition to diabetes also worsen the chance of getting seriously ill from COVID-19, because the body's ability to fight off infection is compromised. The ADA also suggested that if diabetics develop COVID-19 symptoms such as fever, dry cough, and shortness of breath, they should immediately contact their doctor and have glucose readings available for review. Also keep track of fluid consumption, keep a clear list of symptoms, and be sure to ask questions on how to manage diabetes while enduring COVID-19.

Shipping on certain items was delayed during the pandemic. However, leading manufacturers of insulin and diabetic supplies reported that COVID-19 was not affecting the impact of manufacturing and distribution capabilities. The ADA has resources to help if diabetics are struggling to pay for insulin or know someone who is and suggest visiting the website insulinhelp.org for more information.

Your regional physicians are here for you if you need us during this or any health crisis. We hope you won't.

REFERENCES

1 CDC updates, expands list of people at risk of severe COVID-19 illness. Centers for Disease Control and Prevention, June 25, 2020. https://www.cdc.gov/media/releases/2020/p0625-update-expands -COVID-19.html.
2 How COVID-19 impacts people with diabetes. American Diabetes Association. https://diabetes.org/coronavirus-covid-19/how-coronavirus -impacts-people-with-diabetes. Accessed August 30, 2022.

# 17

## Substance Use Disorder during COVID

### CLAY ANDERSON

*Editor's Note: The pandemic's effects on people reckoning up how we lived our lives caused varying motivations. Some wanted to leave addiction; others began self-medicating with nonprescribed drugs or abused prescriptions as a coping medication for the trauma of the times in which we live. Much remains to be studied about how the substance use disorder community fared and what resources they will need to recover from postpandemic trauma, but this chapter includes statistics and analysis of what was known at the time.*

What happens to people with substance use disorder when their lifeline of interpersonal connectedness is placed in jeopardy by a global pandemic? The novel coronavirus called for all Americans to isolate. Could anything be more important for public health—or worse for someone suffering substance abuse disorder?

The following is an anonymous personal story of what active addiction was like for one opioid user during the pandemic. I'm not going to offer any context on how I know this person. He is male, from Appalachia, and now in recovery. That will have to do.

A FIRST-PERSON ACCOUNT OF OPIOID ADDICTION,
AS SHARED WITH THE AUTHOR

*I never intended to become an addict when I started using drugs at 13 years old. I never had a clue that I would become physically* dependent on a drug in such a short amount of time, that my thinking and behavior would change so drastically, that I would lose loving relationships with family and friends, and that I would become unemployable and eventually homeless and penniless.

I was raised to know the difference between right and wrong, to respect others and their property, and to be kind and courteous to others no matter how they treated me in return. I grew up in a loving and safe home and by accounts had a normal childhood. I played sports and made good grades in school. Everyone I knew loved me. The problem was, I did not love myself. During adolescence I formed a negative self-image and was never comfortable in my own skin. I grew anxious and depressed and did not know how to ask for help.

I just wanted to escape the thoughts and feelings I had, which were in part responsible for the comfort and escapism I found in drugs, specifically opioids. I started hanging out with the wrong crowd and experimenting with drugs and alcohol: it provided the escape that I was looking for. Opioids were the catalyst to my bottom. I found opioids at age 17, and after three years of use they brought me to the absolute depths of despair.

In the beginning when I would use opioids, I felt mentally calm, and the incessant chatter between my ears was silenced. I felt like I was wrapped in a warm blanket, and the cares of the world would just slip away. I felt at home in my own skin for the first time in years. It also gave me this amazing energy that I had not felt in years. I remember thinking, "This is what normal people must feel like all the time."

It took about three months of daily use. I found that I would wake up anxious, sweating, and before I could even fathom going to work or doing what other productive members of society did in a day, I had to use opioids to feel normal. By this time in my addiction, I needed it just to function. It was the first thing I thought of upon awakening. Opioids became my primary motivation of the day, surpassing all other basic necessities of life. I was driven by what I call "the autopilot."

On any given day, I had every intention of just doing enough opioids to get me through the day. It never seemed to work out that way. I found myself at my dealer's house, sometimes wondering how I got there. It was like the car drove itself. I had no control over my use.

*Finding ways and means to get more opioids became a 24-hour-per-day job. I could not stop trying because I knew the sickness was coming. If I had to lie, cheat, and steal, I would. At first, I knew better and would try to sell something I owned. When all that was gone, it was either steal or be sick. At the time I would do just about anything to keep from being sick. The sickness of acute withdrawal from opioids is the worst thing I have ever experienced in my life. Withdrawal is so mentally, emotionally, and physically taxing that death would be a relief. Every second was like an eternity. I would sweat profusely from every pore in my body but at the same time be freezing, no matter how warm it was. I had the endless need to move my legs so I would not have to shake my whole body. There was a terrible pain that emanated from every bone in my body. It felt like my bones were breaking from the inside out. Then came the vomiting and diarrhea. If I could have crawled out of my skin, I would have. I had constant thoughts and feelings of guilt, shame, and fear that only abated when I got the opioids in my body. The insomnia was the icing on the cake. There are 86,400 seconds in a day. There were many days when I counted all of them. During one attempt at detox at the age of 19, I went over nine days without one moment of sleep.*

*To nonaddicts, the insanity of drug addiction is hard to fathom. I still cannot believe some of the things I did to get drugs. If I heard that someone had opioids that made people overdose, that is the stuff I would seek out. I remember thinking, "At least there is comfort there: that would be the way I would want to leave this world."*

*At the end of my using, I ended up homeless and penniless with an opioid habit to support. I was utterly and completely isolated, and that is a very dangerous place for an addict to be. At that point, I was under the complete control of a drug and had a mental autopilot driving me that had only one destination: opioids. Somehow, somewhere, a light shone through and I was open for help. "Please, please, please, I cannot live like this anymore!" Luckily for me, someone was there. Others are not so lucky. Of the six friends I went to high school and started using opioids with, three are dead from overdoses. If I had not jumped at that opportunity for help, I knew the autopilot was*

*going to kick in and I would be off trying to get comfortable, with no
regard about who I had to hurt.*

*What worked for me in my recovery process was and is a biosocial approach. Interpersonal connectedness to others was necessary
for every stage. I needed help through the physical and mental withdrawals that I got from my connection with the medical community
in the form of medication-assisted therapy. I needed others who had
walked this path of recovery to show me how to do it: I found this
connection in the rooms of a 12-step program.*

## THE NEUROBIOLOGICAL BASIS OF ADDICTION

Neuroscience research has revealed that addiction is a chronic, relapsing disease of the brain triggered by repeated exposure to drugs
in those who are vulnerable. Addiction is characterized by the loss
of control over drug intake, high motivation to obtain the drug of
choice (or any drug, at a certain point), and a persistent craving for
the drug.[1]

No one knows who will become addicted when an individual
experiments with drugs. The risk for drug addiction is complex and
based upon the interactions between biological and environmental factors. Biological factors such as genetics account for approximately half of the risk for addiction.[2] Environmental factors such as
social and cultural systems, stress, and trauma have been shown to
increase susceptibility to addiction as well. Early life stress can influence the development of the hypothalamic-pituitary-adrenal (HPA)
axis, leading to increased reactivity to stress and susceptibility to
addiction.[3] The HPA is your body's central stress response system,
hooking your central nervous and endocrine systems to each other
in a perpetual cycle of mutual care and information sharing.

Adolescents are often seen as more likely than adults to experiment with drugs and to develop substance use disorders. This understanding in part reflects the fact that the adolescent brain has not
completed its development and is more adaptive to changes than
the adult brain. The human brain continues to develop until the
early to mid-20s; the rate of development differs across neuronal

circuits, with development occurring faster for reward/motivation and emotional circuits than for circuits involved in executive functioning, like judgment, logic, and reasoning. These executive functions are among the last to develop. As a result, during adolescence, the reward/motivation and emotional circuits are hyperactive, leading to greater emotional reactivity and reward-seeking behaviors. Moreover, the executive functioning areas cannot fully self-regulate, leading to more impulsivity and risk taking.[4] Early exposure to drugs of abuse may further impair the development of the executive functioning areas, increasing the long-term risk for addiction.[5] The increased ability of the adolescent brain to adapt and change explains why addiction develops faster in an adolescent than in an adult,[6] and it also explains the greater sensitivity of adolescents to environmental stimuli, such as stress, that influence drug taking.[3]

About half of those who end up addicted to drugs start out as a social user without the intention to become addicted. (The other half get prescriptions, also without intent to become addicted.) However, repeated exposure to the drug activates a primal pathological relationship with a neurotransmitter surge in their brain at the expense of other relationships in their lives. Addiction affects primal behavioral control centers of the brain that operate in large part under the control of a neurotransmitter called dopamine.[1] Other neurotransmitters are also implicated in the formation of addiction, but dopamine is the principal neurotransmitter involved.

Dopamine has many functions in the brain, including the modulation and control of behavior. It modulates reward to stimuli, such as telling us that chocolate is good, therefore motivating us to ingest chocolate. When this reward/motivation pathway is pathological, it results in addiction.[1] The symptoms of addiction are behavioral: movement disorders such as Parkinson's, and mood disorders producing psychoses such as abnormal behavior, delusions, and hallucinations.

Opioids and other drugs cause an extreme surge in the dopamine reward system in the brain. This dopamine system modulates memory and judgment as well. The drugs hijack this primal system responsible for telling us that we are experiencing pleasurable things like food and sex. And this dopamine increase is reinforced with continued use, causing structural changes in the brain. As a result, the reward circuit's capacity to respond to reward and motivate actions that are not drug related is decreased. The things that were once considered pleasurable, like participation in sports and relationships with loved ones, fall secondary to the intense dopamine surge that drugs such as opioids cause. Additionally, the sensitivity of the emotional circuits to stress is enhanced, and the capacity to self-regulate is impaired. The area in the brain responsible for logic, judgment, and reasoning becomes less able to inhibit the reward system's stranglehold on behavior. The result is compulsive drug seeking and taking despite a strong desire to quit.[2]

Drug addiction produces a cycle of drug consumption, "the intoxication phase," drug craving, and drug withdrawal. Either the cycle is broken and the individual enters recovery or drug consumption reoccurs. Relapse is a common occurrence in addiction. Physical withdrawal, negative emotional states, and craving for the drug all produce a strong behavioral drive for drug taking.

During the intoxication phase, the drug stimulates large bursts of dopamine that contribute to the pleasurable or euphoric responses and to the changes in the brain that result in addiction.[7] Secondly, large bursts of dopamine in the reward system reinforce drug taking and strengthen conditioned associations (stimuli that precede drug consumption linked with the expectation of reward), or drug cues.[8,9] Counterintuitively, in a person suffering from addiction, the drug-induced dopamine increases are lessened and the same level of intoxication requires more and more of the drug to achieve the desired effect.[10]

Craving and drug cues themselves elicit dopamine release, triggering the motivation to seek and consume the drug.[11] This phase shows a decrease in the executive control areas of the brain, which are responsible for inhibiting unwanted behaviors and increases in circuits that underlie the increase value of drug taking, as well as circuits that mediate conditioned responses.[12,13] There is heightened sensitivity and reactivity to cues and to adverse emotions that trigger the urgent motivation for and preoccupation with drug taking.[14] This essentially describes the autopilot mechanism that was mentioned in our opening story.

The withdrawal phase is associated with negative mood, anhedonia (inability to experience pleasure), increased sensitivity to stress, and significant dysphoria and anxiety. Such a response is typically observed in an individual with a longer drug exposure history. The duration of exposure needed for a response to emerge varies for the different types of drugs: opioids produce these effects particularly rapidly. Increased signaling in these circuits triggers aversive symptoms that render the individual vulnerable to cravings and preoccupation with taking the drug as means to counteract this aversive state.[3]

In a brain not affected by addiction, the circuits controlling desire for a drug are held in check by underlying executive function areas, which also support making rational, healthy decisions, and that regulate emotions. Thus, the awareness that a drug will provide an immediate reward is balanced by consideration of long-term goals, and the individual is able to make a reasonable choice and carry it through. However, when the underlying executive functions are hypofunctional—as a result of repeated drug exposure or from an underlying vulnerability—and the underlying conditioned responses and stress reactivity are hyperactive—as a result of drug withdrawal and long-term changes in the brain that decrease sensitivity to nondrug rewards—the addicted individual is at a tremendous disadvantage in opposing the strong motivation to take the drug. This explains the difficulty addicted individuals face when trying to stop taking drugs even when they experience negative consequences and have become tolerant to the drug's pleasurable effects. The changes in the brain responsible for these maladaptive behaviors can persist for months or even years after drug discontinuation, but they are amenable to treatment.[3]

WHEN THE DRUG EPIDEMIC AND THE CORONAVIRUS PANDEMIC COLLIDE

Isolation caused by the coronavirus pandemic increases tragic results such as emergency medical service (EMS) calls, emergency department (ED) visits, and overdoses for individuals suffering from addiction, especially opioid addiction. Isolation due to lockdowns, stay-at-home orders, and social distancing serves as a catalyst to make outcomes worse for those individuals.

The drug epidemic in the United States has been ongoing for decades. One of the drugs at the center of this epidemic is opioids, either prescribed or illicit. In 2019 the National Safety Council reported that for the first time, Americans were more likely to die from an accidental opioid overdose than in a motor vehicle wreck.[15] More than 750,000 people died from a drug overdose in the United States from 1999 to 2018,[16] with nearly 450,000 deaths involving prescribed or illicit opioids.[17] Recent yearly estimates indicate that the overdose epidemic peaked in 2017, with 70,723 reported deaths.[18] Although progress has been made overall, fentanyl-related deaths threaten to bring deaths from drug overdoses to tragic new heights. The 12-month rolling count of provisional overdose deaths associated with nonmethadone synthetic opioids (likely fentanyl) increased every month since at least January 2015 (5,766 overdose deaths) through December 2019 (36,509 overdose deaths).[18]

The CDC describes the opioid epidemic as having three waves. The first opioid wave began in the 1990s due to the push toward using opioid medications for chronic pain management and the increased promotion by pharmaceutical companies for medical professionals to use their opioid medications.[19] The second wave of the opioid epidemic started around 2010 and was characterized by the rise in heroin use and overdose deaths.[20] The third wave of the opioid epidemic began in 2013. This wave coincides with the steep rise in overdose deaths that involved synthetic opioids, particularly illegally produced fentanyl.[5] Fentanyl is a highly potent synthetic opioid, even at extremely low doses. An amount about the size of a few grains of salt is enough to kill most people. Opioids work in the brain to produce a variety of effects; however, they all act as central nervous system depressants. The fatal effect is the decrease in how often and how deeply one breathes, which causes a mismatch between how much oxygen is in the blood to supply the body's demands to function and survive.

Nora D. Volkow, MD, director of the National Institute on Drug Abuse (part of the National Institutes of Health), explained, "We do not yet have nationwide data that capture the full impact of COVID-19 and its related societal effects on overdose deaths, but some indicators show troubling increases associated with it."[21]

The CDC provisional drug overdose death count, updated through April 2020, showed an increase in overdose deaths.[21] The overdose detection mapping application program (ODMAP) data is a surveillance system that provides near real-time suspected overdose data. Collected from law enforcement agencies, fire departments, emergency medical services, hospitals, and medical examiners, ODMAP data shows a 17.59 percent increase in suspected overdoses following the enactment of stay-at-home orders.[21,22] Nationally, suspected overdose submissions to ODMAP in 2020 rose by 18 percent in March, 29 percent in April, and 42 percent in May, based on a 30-day rolling mean comparison to these months in 2019.[16] The ODMAP report showed increases of 11.4 percent for fatal overdoses and 18.6 percent for nonfatal overdoses during 2020.[23]

Volkow called these trends "absolutely concerning" and correlational with reports of increased substance use of all types.[21] A study that analyzed changes in clinical drug testing patterns and results at a national clinical laboratory compared data obtained before and during the pandemic. The study analyzed 872,762 urine specimens from all 50 states and the District of Columbia as part of clinical drug testing performed from January 1, 2019, through May 16, 2020. The COVID-19 pandemic time period included specimens tested March 15 to May 16.

The data suggested that nonprescribed fentanyl increased by 35 percent during the pandemic compared to the baseline period. In the same period, nonprescribed heroin increased by 44 percent, other opiates increased by 10 percent, and marijuana increased by 4 percent.[23]

Another concerning fact discovered by the study was that the combination of nonprescribed fentanyl with other drugs also increased during the pandemic. Some drug dealers are mixing fentanyl with drugs such as heroin, cocaine, methamphetamine, and ecstasy. This is because it takes very little to produce a high with fentanyl, making it a cheaper option. That becomes especially risky when people taking drugs don't realize they might contain fentanyl as a cheap but dangerous additive. They might be taking stronger opioids than their bodies are used to and thus be more likely to overdose.[24] Specifically, positivity for nonprescribed fentanyl increased by 89 percent among patients positive for amphetamines; 48 percent for individuals with benzodiazepines; 34 percent for individuals positive for cocaine; 39 percent for other opiates; and 4 percent for heroin.[23]

Ayana Jordan, MD, assistant professor and addiction psychiatrist at the Yale University School of Medicine, did not find the increase in overdoses over the pandemic surprising. She pointed to the "increased isolation, financial duress of loved ones and despair people are facing" as significant risk factors.[21]

Addiction Policy Forum conducted a survey to better understand the impact of COVID-19 on individuals with a substance use disorder. They found 4 percent of respondents nationwide reported an overdose since the pandemic began. Family member substance use had changed because of COVID-19 according to 24 percent of respondents, with 20 percent reporting increased substance use.[6]

HAS THE APPALACHIAN REGION BEEN
UNIQUELY AFFECTED DURING THE PANDEMIC?

The Appalachian region has been considered an epicenter of the opioid crisis since its inception. Statistics only begin to tell the story of its destruction in real lives. By 2011, the Appalachian region overdose mortality rate was five times as high as the rate in 1999. And in 2011, the overdose mortality rate in the Appalachian region was 64 percent higher than non-Appalachian states, climbing to 65 percent higher in 2015 before dropping to 48 percent in 2018. Opioid-related overdose death data in 2018 showed that opioids caused 4,548 deaths in the Appalachia region.[25]

Anecdotal evidence has suggested dramatic increases in overdose deaths in many regions during the COVID-19 pandemic. Not only does everyone know someone who has died of COVID at this point, but most of us have lost someone due to substance abuse. The impact of COVID-19 will likely lead to an increase in mortality, particularly as the Appalachian region and the rest of the United States experience isolation, economic challenges as a result of the pandemic, and limitations on access to in-person treatment and recovery support.[25]

Statistics from the West Virginia Department of Health and Human Resources show that emergency room visits related to overdoses were higher in June, July, and August 2020 than they were during the same months in 2019.[22]

Hospital-presenting opioid overdoses reported to the Tennessee Department of Health from January 2020 to October 2020 were up 65 percent compared to the previous time frame in 2019. Since the onset of the pandemic in March 2020, overdoses in Tennessee spiked in May and June before declining to 2019 levels in October. Actual opioid overdoses from January 2020 to October 2020 were 7,213 compared to 4,706 in the same time frame for 2019. The entire 2019 year had approximately 5,906. Each month of 2020 has surpassed its 2019 month by comparison, with the exception of October 2020.[26]

Preliminary data from the Virginia Department of Health, focused on the four southwestern health districts from March through October 2020, showed a 26 percent increase in opioid-related drug overdose deaths compared to the same time frame from the previous year. The actual number of deaths was 110 persons. This is 10 percent greater than the peak opioid-related drug overdose deaths occurring in 2017.[27]

I conducted an interview with an emergency medical technician with ten years of experience in southwestern Virginia. He said, "Before COVID, opioid overdoses were in the back of my mind every day when I would go into the field. Now, during the COVID pandemic, I expect to see an opioid overdose every day when I go into the field."

A study that evaluated the changes in the average daily Kentucky EMS opioid overdose runs conducted between January 14, 2020, and April 26, 2020 (52 days before and after the COVID-19 state of emergency declaration, March 6, 2020) found that daily runs increased after the COVID-19 state emergency declaration. There was a 17 percent increase in the number of EMS opioid overdose runs with transportation to an emergency department, a 71 percent increase in runs with refused transportation, and a 50 percent increase in runs for suspected opioid overdoses with deaths at the scene. The average daily EMS opioid overdose runs with refused transportation increased significantly, doubling to an average of eight opioid overdose patients refusing transportation every day during the COVID-related study period.[28]

### CONTRIBUTING FACTORS AND OPTIONS TO COUNTER THEM

Addiction is a chronic disease, so its treatment should follow a sustained model of intervention, the intensity of which should be adjusted to the stage of the disease.[2] Social isolation and stress during the pandemic exacerbate the lack of or disruption in medical services, contributing to the results that have been presented here.

Stress, change, job losses, loneliness, and depression can all trigger prescription medication overuse, illicit drug use, and relapses of drug abuse.[29] Notably, social distancing during the COVID-19 pandemic has isolated vulnerable patients, leaving them to misuse prescription or illicit drugs alone. Volkow was among those who noted that isolation drives people to initiate drug taking or to relapse.[30]

Making matters worse, some treatment centers have been forced to close or scale back significantly during the pandemic shutdowns, leaving less access to those individuals who are actively seeking help or are in a substance use treatment center vulnerable to a lack or disruption in the vital services they need.[4,31] A survey by the Addictions Policy Forum reported that more than a third (34 percent) of the respondents had experienced disruptions accessing treatment or recovery support since the start of the pandemic, and 14 percent said they were unable to obtain needed services.[6]

Isolation removes the support system that individuals suffering from addiction desperately need. Interpersonal connectedness is the antidote to decrease fatalities for those suffering with addiction, especially opioid addiction, whether it is connection with family when reaching out for help, getting into a drug treatment facility, with peers at 12-step meetings that are experiencing similar hardships, or with their medical provider for medication-assisted therapy.

In short, if you love someone who has an addiction, call them. Check in on them. Help them access vaccine boosters when they are eligible. Get them back into the community. The opposite of addiction is connection.

### REFERENCES

1 Yager, L.M., Garcia, A.F., Wunsch, A.M., Ferguson, S.M. The ins and outs of the striatum: role in drug addiction. *Neuroscience,* June 23, 2015. National Library of Medicine. https://pubmed.ncbi.nlm.nih.gov/26116518/.

2 Volkow, N.D., Michaelides, M., Baler, R. The neuroscience of drug reward and addiction. *Physiological Reviews.* 2019;99(4):2115–2140. doi:10.1152/physrev.00014.2018.

3 Volkow, N.D., Boyle, M., Stahre. M. Neuroscience of addiction: relevance to prevention and treatment. *American Journal of Psychiatry.* 2018;175(8):729–740. doi:10.1176/appi.ajp.2018.17101174.

4 Volkow, N.D. Addressing the unique challenges of COVID-19 for people in recovery. National Institute on Drug Abuse, November 19, 2020. nida.nih.gov/about-nida/noras-blog/2020/09/addressing-unique-challenges-covid-19-people-in-recovery.

5 Gladden, R.M., Martinez, P., Seth, P. Fentanyl law enforcement submissions and increases in synthetic opioid-involved overdose deaths—27 States, 2013–2014. Center for Disease Control and Prevention, August 17, 2017. https://www.cdc.gov/mmwr/volumes/65/wr/mm6533a2.htm.

6 Hulsey, J., Mellis, A., Kelly, B. COVID-19 pandemic impact on patients, families and individuals in recovery from substance use disorders. Addiction Policy Forum, May 2020. https://www.addictionpolicy.org/covid19-report.

7 Potenza, M.N., Sofuoglu, M., Carroll, K.M., Rounsaville, B.J. Neuroscience of behavioral and pharmacological treatments for addictions. *Neuron.* 2011;69(4):695–712. doi:10.1016/j.neuron.2011.02.009.

8 Di Chiara, G. Nucleus accumbens shell and core dopamine: differential role in behavior and addiction. *Behavioral Brain Research.* 2002;137(1–2):75–114. doi:10.1016/S0166-4328(02)00286-3.

9  Volkow, N.D., Baler, R.D. NOW vs LATER brain circuits: implications for obesity and addiction. *Trends in Neurosciences.* 2015;38(6):345–352. doi:10.1016/j.tins.2015.04.002.
10 Volkow, N.D., Wang, G., Fowler, J.S., Tomasi, D., Telang, F., Baler, R. Addiction: decreased reward sensitivity and increased expectation sensitivity conspire to overwhelm the brain's control circuit. *BioEssays.* 2010;32(9):748–755. doi:10.1002/bies.201000042.
11 Volkow, N.D., Wang, G., Telang, F., et al. Cocaine cues and dopamine in dorsal striatum: mechanism of craving in cocaine addiction. *Journal of Neuroscience.* 2006;26(24):6583–6588. doi:10.1523/JNEUROSCI.1544-06.2006.
12 Volkow, N.D., Wang, G., Telang, F., et al. Activation of orbital and medial prefrontal cortex by methylphenidate in cocaine-addicted subjects but not in controls: relevance to addiction. *Journal of Neuroscience.* 2005;25(15):3932–3939. doi:10.1523/JNEUROSCI.0433-05.2005.
13 Robbins, T.W., Ersche K.D., Everitt, B.J. Drug addiction and the memory systems of the brain. *Annals of the New York Academy of Sciences.* 2008;1141:1–21. doi:10.1196/annals.1441.020.
14 Volkow, N.D., Koob, G.F., McLellan, A.T. Neurobiologic advances from the brain disease model of addiction. *New England Journal of Medicine.* 2016;374:363–371. doi:10.1056/NEJMra1511480.
15 For the first time, we're more likely to die from accidental opioid overdose than motor vehicle crash. National Safety Council, January 14, 2019. https://www.nsc.org/in-the-newsroom/for-the-first-time-were-more-likely-to-die-from-accidental-opioid-overdose-than-motor-vehicle-crash.
16 Data overview: the drug overdose epidemic: behind the numbers. Centers for Disease Control and Prevention, December 7, 2020. https://www.cdc.gov/drugoverdose/data/index.html.
17 Hedegaard, H., Miniño, A.M., Warner, M. Drug overdose deaths in the United States, 1999–2018. NCHS data brief no. 356. Centers for Disease Control and Prevention, January 30, 2020. https://www.cdc.gov/nchs/products/databriefs/db356.htm.
18 Wilson, N., Kariisa, M., Seth, P., Smith, H., Davis, N.L. Drug and opioid-involved overdose deaths—United States, 2017–2018. Centers for Disease Control and Prevention, March 19, 2020. https://www.cdc.gov/mmwr/volumes/69/wr/mm6911a4.htm.
19 Guideline for opioids for chronic (1). Scribd. https://www.scribd.com/document/393870560/Guideline-for-Opioids-for-Chronic-1. Accessed June 15, 2022.

20 Understanding the epidemic. Centers for Disease Control and Prevention, March 19, 2020. https://www.cdc.gov/drugoverdose/epidemic/index.html.

21 Gold, J. Overdoses are increasing in the U.S. over COVID-19: here's what addiction experts want you to know. *Forbes,* December 15, 2020. https://www.forbes.com/sites/jessicagold/2020/12/14/overdoses-are-increasing-in-the-us-over-covid-19-heres-what-addiction-experts-want-you-to-know/?sh=65445ebc4ffa.

22 Patterson, B., Lofton, K., Marema, T. Has COVID-19 led to an increase in substance use disorders? 100 Days in Appalachia, November 2, 2020. https://www.100daysinappalachia.com/2020/10/has-covid-19-led-to-an-increase-in-substance-use-disorders/.

23 "Understanding the Epidemic." Centers for Disease Control and Prevention, March 19, 2020. https://www.cdc.gov/drugoverdose/epidemic/index.html.

24 Niles, J.K., Gudin, J., Radcliff, J., Kaufman, H.W. The opioid epidemic within the COVID-19 pandemic: drug testing in 2020. Mary Ann Liebert, October 8, 2020. doi:10.1089/pop.2020.0230.

25 Meit, M. Appalachian diseases of despair. Appalachian Regional Commission, November 19, 2020. https://www.arc.gov/report/appalachian-diseases-of-despair/.

26 Facts & figures. Tennessee Department of Health. https://www.tn.gov/health/health-program-areas/pdo/pdo/facts-figures. Accessed June 15, 2022.

27 Rosner, J. Interview by author, December 11, 2020.

28 Slavova, S., Rock, P., Bush, H.M., Quesinberry, D., Walsh, S.L. Signal of increased opioid overdose during COVID-19 from emergency medical services data. *Drug and Alcohol Dependence.* 2020;214:108–176. doi:10.1016/j.drugalcdep.2020.108176.

29 Sinha, R. How does stress increase risk of drug abuse and relapse? *Psychopharmacology.* 2001;158:343–359. doi:10.1007/s002130100917.

30 Collins, F. Coping with the collision of public health crises: COVID-19 and substance use disorders. National Institutes of Health; U.S. Department of Health and Human Services, April 21, 2020. https://directorsblog.nih.gov/2020/04/21/coping-with-the-collision-of-public-health-crises-covid-19-and-substance-use-disorders/.

31 Giles, B. Coronavirus crisis disrupts treatment for another epidemic: addiction. *Los Angeles Times,* July 6, 2020. https://www.latimes.com/science/story/2020-07-06/coronavirus-crisis-disrupts-addiction-treatment.

# 18

## The Race to Vaccinate

### RAKESH PATEL

*Editor's Note: By the time vaccines began to roll out in late 2020, the politics of American responses to COVID made clear the longed-for end would not come easily. Endemic replaced pandemic as pundits debated themes of personal rights versus public good. Touted by many as the protection that would return us to normalcy, vaccines became conspiracy theory fodder for others. The frustration of the medical community toward misinformation, tempered by respect for patient wishes, comes out in Dr. Patel's first-person account of his encounters with sincere mistrust. How does a doctor combat false information when patients are unwilling to even ask questions?*

In November 2019, my wife and I took a vacation to Thailand. Our lengthy return to the USA included a long layover in China. We had the option of remaining in the airport but stumbled on the concept of "layover tours." For about $100 you could book an eight-hour tour of the Great Wall of China. This included a private vehicle operated by an English-speaking driver picking you up from the airport. The cab dropped you at Mutianyu, located just outside of Beijing, where you could complete a self-tour of the ancient frontier walls.

Of course, this was all prepandemic, and we thought a Great Wall visit would be a wonderful way to make use of our time. The tour was excellent, and the monument was spectacular. We were not rushed to get back to the airport. The memories remain pleasant and an unexpected highlight of our trip. We had no idea that would be the last time we indulged our love for travel for a couple of years. A few short months after our return to the USA, the medical community here in America learned about the novel coronavirus that was initially thought to have begun in a seafood market in Wuhan, China.

On January 19, 2020, a 35-year-old male presented to an urgent care center in Snohomish County in Washington with a four-day cough and shortness of breath. He did not smoke. His physical examination revealed rhonchus, a rattling sound made while breathing, caused by secretions or fluid in the lungs. Rhonchi often indicates a wet lung from infection or fluid that is difficult to clear, yet his chest X-rays were normal. Next came an extensive panel of respiratory infection tests, including influenza, adenovirus, rhinovirus, and respiratory syncytial virus—which were all negative.

Given his travel history, the US Department of Health was notified, which in turn reached out to the Centers for Disease Control Emergency Operations Center. The agencies all agreed that the patient should undergo testing for COVID-19. His test was confirmed to be positive on January 20, prompting his admission to an airborne isolation unit at Providence Regional Medical Center for clinical observation. This man became the first documented patient on American soil to test positive for the COVID pandemic.[1] He remained clinically stable, other than occasional fevers and a high heart rate. His symptoms also improved after receiving IV infusion of remdesivir, a novel antiviral drug soon widely used for the treatment of moderate to severe infection in patients that required hospitalization.

He was the first of millions. Midway through June 2021, just over 599,000 of those COVID-19 patients would die of the infection from which he recovered. That same month, the US had reduced its death rates from more than 4,000 to about 300 per day. Worldwide, 176 million reported cases had resulted in 3.1 million confirmed deaths.

These were tragic statistics, masking individual and unique sadness, and yet simultaneously hopeful. The pandemic appeared to be waning.

Many of us are aware that the end of the pandemic is a fuzzy finish line. The end can truly occur only when the virus is no longer prevalent throughout the world's 190+ countries. Dr. Anthony Fauci, now a household name, served as one of many advisers to the US president on when that end can realistically be determined. As a leader in immunology, Fauci predicted that uniting Americans with a considerable degree of diversity within their communities and getting them all to accept vaccination would prove a challenge—let alone doing the same worldwide, and leaving aside unequal access to vaccines in countries with less economic and political clout.

When the first step to ending the pandemic appeared via the development of an effective vaccine, wealthier countries rejoiced as they rolled out vaccine distribution. But the second step in subduing this coronavirus is herd immunity. There are now several vaccines readily available in global communities. On December 31, 2020, the World Health Organization (WHO) issued an emergency use listing (EUL) for the Pfizer-BioNTech (BNT162b2) vaccine. Also that December, the WHO issued use for the Moderna vaccine. On February 15, 2021, an EUL was issued for two versions of the AstraZeneca vaccine and the Ad26 developed by Janssen (Johnson & Johnson) on March 12. First came the race to develop a vaccine, but later we health providers learned the real race lay in administering it to people riddled with doubts, concerns, and in some cases outright conspiracy theories.

When COVID vaccines first rolled out, only health-care employees and forefront workers deemed essential were eligible. This soon expanded to certain populations based on age and occupation, among other factors. Eventually, anyone over the age of 18 could receive a COVID-19 vaccine, with various states lowering the ages for children after the Food and Drug Administration issued guidelines for vaccine administration to youth.

It is terrible to know that we were so unprepared for this pandemic, yet remarkable how quickly the scientific and medical communities were able to develop a vaccine, especially with that development using novel technology. The US government played an integral role in securing billions of dollars to fund research and development and distribution of the vaccines—perhaps part of the reason that the virus itself became so political rather than being seen as a true health crisis.

Social media promoted positive images of vaccination use among health-care employees, as many posted videos or pictures of themselves receiving it. Hashtags such as #ImVaccinated or #IGot-Vaccinated and special frames for profile pictures informed viewers of vaccination appreciation and status.

Unfortunately, social media platforms were also used to share misinformation that has influenced people's decisions against receiving the vaccine. False claims circulating in 2021 included infertility claims (that the vaccine was designed to make everyone, or specific racial and ethnic groups, sterile). There were also allegations that the vaccination would cause DNA changes, involve a microchip to be activated later, or use fetal matter from aborted babies.[2]

Central Appalachia was a particularly targeted and perhaps receptive victim regarding these claims, many of which were astroturfed by specific bad actors; *astroturfing* is when an organization or entity provokes conversation or action by circulating false or misleading information with intent to agitate grassroots responses, often for personal gain.[2] In an online world full of data readily accessible at your fingertips, credibility becomes the major concern. People do not lack good information; they drown in bad intel.

A good source of reliable data during all this confusion should have been primary care providers, especially during unique circumstances, such as infection or pregnancy. Unfortunately, people prone to vaccine hesitancy or medical mistrust might not have such a trusted individual in the first place, or they engage in confirmation bias if they do (looking only for data or conversations that support their existing predilections), lending credence to astroturfed conspiracies circulating in their media feeds.

Researchers at Virginia Tech were among many nationwide who began to investigate online breeding grounds for misinformation plaguing the Appalachian regions. They received a small grant for the study, involving 1,048 study participants across the 13 states represented within Appalachia.[3] Before the study was over, it was reported that almost half of the respondents believed the vaccine could cause infertility; up to 40 percent believed in a high risk of serious side effects, including paralysis. Some viral vaccinations throughout history have on occasion provoked a response commonly referred to as Bell's palsy, a temporary facial paralysis.[4] This droop can often interfere with speech and feeding. Hyping these side effects online with overinflated statistics was a natural move for bad actors intent on agitation and astroturfing.

Sadly, just under 20 percent of Appalachians reported believing that the vaccinations were not real because the coronavirus and pandemic were not real. In some states, respondents referred to "the election virus," implying the crisis was a deliberate attempt to discredit the incumbent president.

The political implications of that nickname show up even more in vaccine hesitancy. A CBS news poll from April 2020 found that 33 percent of Republicans said they would not get the vaccine, compared to 10 percent of Democrats.[5] If there is so much hesitancy for vaccination based on political beliefs, how can it be widely accepted as an important process for pandemic resolution? How can a health crisis transcend politics? Are local governments not reaching various communities; are the concerns of local governments also too politicized to prioritize health? Who watches the watchdogs?

These questions remain largely unanswered, and probably will remain so—which begs the question: What happens the next time a global health crisis emerges?

Another area of concern throughout Appalachia is physical access to health care; put bluntly, one must be in the same room as the professional who administers a shot, at a physical site such as a clinic or pharmacy. As vaccines rolled into rural areas, it was necessary for fairgrounds, grocery stores, and other community-trusted areas to be pressed into service for inoculations. Rural counties have historically struggled with access issues; roads are curvy and narrow and well off the beaten interstate paths. Costs of delivering care to small group populations are higher than in metropolitan areas.

Yet the vaccine held additional, unique challenges. The temperature storage requirements of the vaccines and their limited shelf life once opened create logistical challenges unconsidered prior to the pandemic and not encompassed in urban policy development. Rural challenges are covered in other chapters in this book, including the prepandemic economics that threatened small rural hospitals and the difficulty of workforce development in areas dominated by single hospital systems or lacking hospital access entirely. Suffice it to say, two major factors plagued vaccine rollout in central Appalachia: getting vaccinations to the people and people refusing to get vaccinated.

Resistance to vaccination for COVID-19 has been nationwide, but according to national media reports, geographic distinctions exist in the Midwest and in the South. In fact, an April 2021 article in *Forbes* lists Mississippi and Idaho as the most reticent, at 30 and 29 percent of their state populations, respectively.[6] Overlaying voting maps against the states with the lowest vaccination rates can be equal parts revealing and disturbing. When health is political, bad things follow. Every doctor knows this—whether we can do anything about it or not.

Indeed, the stirring up of controversy over the vaccines seemed to target "hot potato" political issues and themes important to specific voting groups—another signal of the infamous astroturfing. Aborted-fetal-material rumors poured gas on a red-hot flame for pro-lifers. Rumors of sterilization struck fear in communities of color, who have legitimately been victims of targeted involuntary sterilizations, as late as the 1990s for Indigenous women worldwide.[7] America's last awareness of forced sterilization was the late 1970s, well within living memory for women who must now decide for themselves and advise their daughters and grandchildren on COVID vaccination.[8]

To parse those with historic precedent for medical mistrust from those whose values—political, religious, and so on—support specific worldviews would not only be impossible but counterproductive from a medical point of view. Patient compliance, as any resident like myself who has spent the past eight years learning to practice medicine will tell you, rests on a complicated series of interactions. How much does the patient trust the doctor? How much does the doctor trust the patient? What is the patient's cultural background? What kind of access does the patient have to a regular provider with whom they can build a relationship? And on and on the list goes. Suffice it to say, as doctors we learn that the body is a system with specific needs, while the mind is a unique and individualized enigma within that body we must treat. To lose the patient's trust is to lose the patient.

Nowhere was this more evident than at the end of 2020. The USA was in a national lockdown, and despite the holidays, millions of Americans decided to stay at home and respect recommendations for social isolation. If there is an Appalachian value more important than family, I have yet to see it in action. Even though much has been made of the surge of cases experienced regionally from a few days after Thanksgiving through the New Year, I wish to point out that the surge could have been much, much worse. Some people traveled despite the risks. Many did not, and every one of us who lives here, loves here, and practices medicine here wishes to thank you for making that decision. You helped!

In fact, local policies and mandates were so effective in some ways that with all the hand hygiene and social distancing that took place from 2020 to 2021, the annual influenza hardly made a dent in our society; it had record-low statistical presence—a small silver lining in a national cloud, and evidence of effectiveness for those willing to see it.

Still, the overwinter of 2020–21 brought a huge viral burden. Almost exactly a year after the United States captured its first case in the distant state of Washington, Virginia (where I practice) peaked at 7,245 new cases on January 18. By March 3 we saw 383 deaths in a single day. One hesitates to discuss money and death in the same paragraph, yet the two rode side by side in the public's mind—unlike in countries like India, where literal death resulted from economic deprivation, leading to mass migrations from cities back to home villages, and starvation on the way.

Appalachian poverty does not reach the levels of poverty seen in other countries, but food insecurity is not a competitive sport. This pandemic has brought so many radical economic changes that have been disastrous for the Appalachian community. Central Appalachia in particular already suffered from a history of extraction without infrastructure building.

I personally struggled financially when I first moved into the Appalachian hills. I was the sole bread earner for a family that included my wife, two young children, and my parents. My father was finally able to find a job at a local hardware store; in the city where we lived previously, he drove for Uber—a company with no presence here. After more than a year, my wife was hired as a pediatric nurse practitioner, just as the pandemic began. It took her company months to get her credentialed; mere weeks after full employment, she was furloughed. This soon turned into a termination due to the clinic not being able to maintain financial viability. She is one of thousands of health-care workers who, ironically, were furloughed, terminated, or unable to find work during the greatest health-care crisis of our generation.

According to the International Labor Organization, the economic burden of the pandemic included the loss of 114 million jobs by December 2020, closures of indeterminate numbers of family-owned businesses, and for the first time in 20 years a significant increase in US poverty.[9] Accompanying these difficulties came a rise in domestic violence and substance abuse. One interesting statistical finding is that over the last 20 years, US divorces have continued to drop.[10] One might ask: Has the pandemic helped this? Will there be yet another shift in cultural values after the pandemic?

National changes in hospital policies included temperature screening of all employees before allowing them to enter the clinic or hospital, restricted visitations, and new cafeteria rules, such as removal of the always beloved salad bar, plus serving preboxed lunches. Residents in my program who had children suddenly found themselves scrambling to address closed schools and manage the dual responsibilities of their work schedule with children who needed to learn online and be supervised at home. The hits came without warning, literally, as school systems struggled to follow the latest guidance available. Disruption followed disruption.

Then there were the patients. Never mind the salad bar's inconvenience. I still see the faces of those who lost their battles or whose lives were forever altered because of their encounters with the virus that some of their neighbors told them did not exist. I will share three different personal patient experiences that still make my nerves cringe when I think of them. Names have been changed to protect identities.

First up, let's call him "Henry." I had just started my shift. It was 6 a.m., and I was receiving sign-out information from the nightshift resident when we heard a code blue (medical emergency) called on the intercom. We both rushed to the announced room. Once the coronavirus took hold, it became normal practice to keep your protective gear on you or close by, including an N95 respirator mask and a pair of protective eyewear, for this very reason: help was being called for in the COVID unit.

After donning all my appropriate protective gear to look like an astronaut, I walked into the room and found a man in his 70s gasping for air. He was obtunded (meaning in an altered state of consciousness, in this case nearly unresponsive and unable to follow any commands). His oxygen levels were very low; although he had been on oxygen previously, he now needed much more.

The nurse who was also at bedside informed me that Henry had a "do not resuscitate, do not intubate" order in place. This means if he ever went into heart or lung failure, we would not be exhausting heroic measures such as chest compressions or artificial breathing devices to prolong Henry's life. My role was to continue treatment, inform his family of the new changes, and continue supportive care.

As I gathered information, I learned that he had been doing well over the last few days and was actually discharged the day before.

When the ambulance brought Henry home, they found no one there, forcing them to bring him back to the hospital. Apparently, Henry's wife was admitted to the hospital for COVID-19 right before Henry was discharged, and this information had not yet been communicated via the family to the hospital. In fact, she was also in the COVID unit, just a few rooms down from his.

Unfortunately, she suffered from severe dementia, so I was not able to talk to her about his condition and prepare her for the worst. I called the patient's son, who had the medical power of attorney and understood the situation clearly. Henry passed later that day.

Similar in age to Henry was "Mike." Mike was transferred to our facility to seek a higher level of intensive care than was available at another county hospital. Mike had COVID, presenting as double pneumonia. He also had severe adult respiratory distress syndrome, which is a nasty complication of COVID; this diagnosis suggests a poor prognosis. Mike was already on life support, and the ventilator settings were approaching maximal settings available when he was transferred to our hospital. His chances for survival were minimal, and we attempted to transition him to comfort measures, from which point family members can unanimously elect to withdraw all life-sustaining devices. The goal is a peaceful, pain-free passage.

Unfortunately, like Henry, Mike's wife had contracted COVID and was being admitted and treated at another regional facility, where she remained unavailable for an entire week. The next of kin was the patient's son, who was having a terrible time coming to terms with the situation and was not able to make any decisions at the time. So we continued supportive care in the intensive care unit (ICU) the best we could. The cost of care for a patient on life support can be up to $10,000 a day. Finally, Mike's wife was discharged home and we were able to contact her with updates, as well as address goals of care. She was agreeable to a terminal wean. This means turning off all life-supporting devices.

However, she had one condition: that she was able to see Mike one last time. Unfortunately, given her recent infection, she would not be allowed to physically be present in our ICU, but she agreed to participate in a videoconference to say her farewells to her husband. We were fortunate to have the equipment (designated tablet) for this very purpose, but when the time came, far too many technological limitations appeared, such as log-in issues, third-party consultation, and other technical and policy issues.

When the nurse approached me about the delays, we were all frustrated, and I saw a simple solution. Giving her my phone, I asked her to make the video call. Of course, we still had to follow policies and procedures, so we used an application called Doximity, which is Health Insurance Portability and Accountability Act compliant. Hospital/ICU administration also needed to approve the use of a personal device to assist in patient care.

We received the green light within minutes, and Mike's diligent and compassionate ICU nurse hosted the conference for his wife, son, and other family members to see and talk to him for as long as they wanted. After all the final words had been said, we turned off life support and provided Mike with IV morphine and oxygen. He passed within minutes. While this was a difficult time for everyone, my guts still wrench when I think of Mike's wife and son, paying their last tributes via a tiny screen and not being able to hold their loved one's hand.

Third and last, I remember "John." I see both John and his wife in my clinic as regular patients. While doctors never have favorite patients, if we did, John's wife would be one of mine. John is in his 80s and has a history of bipolar, dementia, and thyroid disease, all of which can adversely affect mental activity. His wife also has dementia.

John first called the clinic to report fever, persistent coughing, and dark, foul-smelling urine. We conducted a telehealth appointment due to the pandemic. He was difficult to speak with because of his confusion, and he sounded ill. We suspected he had a COVID-19 infection and offered him testing at the clinic the next day. At the time, any patient with respiratory symptoms had to be screened vigorously. Many were given the opportunity to have telehealth appointments, and we conducted drive-by COVID testing once our clinic received the equipment.

John arrived the next day in a vehicle with his wife and two daughters. He was one of the first patients to receive the nasopharyngeal swab and be tested on our new machine. As suspected, he tested positive. Since his symptoms were mild, we asked him to self-isolate at home and scheduled him for an IV infusion of bamlanivimab, one of the first therapies available for patients not sick enough to be admitted to the hospital.

It was and is standard policy that patients who come to our emergency room and test positive for COVID but have mild symptoms are asked to return to their homes and isolate. This frees up hospital beds for more ill patients. While John was not terribly impacted by COVID-19, I suspected that his entire family was affected. His wife also had respiratory symptoms but tested negative several times.

Both John and his wife were able to avoid hospitalization and dodged the complications of COVID. I wanted to share this story to highlight that elderly people with several medical conditions who got COVID could sometimes survive it. He was fortunate. I also wanted to share his story because John does not believe to this day that the vaccination offers any protection, and he does not feel with certainty that it is safe for him. He has never had the seasonal flu vaccine and he continues to refuse the COVID-19 vaccination.

When I graduated from medical school and was awarded my medical diploma, I swore the Hippocratic oath. This is one of the oldest binding documents pledged by physicians to uphold several ethical standards. These include to do no harm, to prevent and treat disease where possible, to respect privacy, but also to respect an individual's choices and decisions in their own care, even when science and provider advice say to do the opposite. This means that I must respect John's decisions about the vaccination regardless of how he supports his choices, and I will continue to care for him. Perhaps I may also continue to discuss the vaccine with him, but the choice is his. Trust between patient and provider includes discerning when to speak and when to listen.

Being at the forefront of this pandemic, I have learned a wealth of information that has contributed to my medical knowledge, clinical practice, outlook, values, and my spiritual and internal growth. It has been an unfortunate learning curve, to be sure, but nevertheless an effective one that involved holistic thinking about how medicine works in society. While social isolation had to be the key ingredient in fighting this pandemic, it came at a high cost of negative social and economic impact. The US government estimated that spending on this pandemic in fiscal year 2020 amounted to $6.5 trillion, which included health research and funding, but also $2.6 trillion for stimulus spending and $900 billion for stimulus tax relief programs.[11]

And so we return to where we started: how to end the pandemic and bring the economy and our social interactions into a new normal. Cleveland Clinic reports that achieving 33–44 percent of vaccinations in a population is adequate to reach herd immunity for the flu, while in contrast 70–85 percent is the estimated requirement for COVID-19.[12] As of May 2021, the US government had issued 291 million vaccinations to people. President Joe Biden's oft-repeated goal of 70 percent of the population having received at least one shot by July 4 was within tantalizing reach. The *Wall Street Journal* reported that the peak of more than 3 million vaccinations per day in April slowed to roughly half that in June 2021. The reason for the slow-down was increasingly attributed to hesitancy rather than access.[13]

This meant that we still had a way to go, and hesitancy rather than access was the dominant delaying factor. Overcoming access obstacles and clarifying misinformation is helpful, and so is getting creative. Some states engaged in highly competitive strategies to win this race. People vaccinated after a certain date were put into a jackpot lottery drawing in a few states. California reportedly gave away the largest pot of prize money: ten Californians were to win $1.5 million each. Maryland offered winners $40,000 a day for 40 days. New Mexico reportedly picked a single jackpot winner to be awarded $5 million.

Finally, I must address what some might choose to call entitled hubris when it comes to vaccination. That is not my choice of wording for this strange situation. Suffice it to say, while Americans refused vaccines, as was their right, other countries desperate to vaccinate their populations begged for access.

Perhaps a story might assist in explaining just how strange and politicized the American vaccine rollout became. In December 2020, a doctor in Houston was fired for distribution of 10 COVID vaccinations that were approaching expiration. Dr. Hasan Gokal, an immigrant to the US, earned his medical degree from SUNY Upstate Medical University in Syracuse, went to work for the Harris County Public Health Department in Texas, and became medical director for its COVID response team. At a public event, a nurse opened a new packet of vaccine doses just before the site closed for the day, leaving 10 that would expire within six hours.

Gokal tried to find someone at the event who needed vaccinating; this included staff, paramedics, and law enforcement agents, all of whom either refused or said they had already been vaccinated. He took the doses home and started calling anyone he knew from his community and neighborhood. After a long evening assisted by his wife, he was able to administer vaccinations to qualified elderly individuals whom he did not intimately know and were plagued by several medical conditions. With 10 minutes to go before expiry, he administered the final dose to his wife (who expressed concern he would get in trouble for doing so).

The following day he submitted the requisite paperwork to the vaccination administration. Although Dr. Gokal followed all the guidelines and protocols, he was later fired for his actions. Soon after he received criminal charges for stealing vaccinations and using his position to administer vaccines in his neighborhood. As of May 2021, a misdemeanor judge had dismissed the case, while a magistrate determined sufficient probable cause to indict. The district attorney in Harris County did not immediately bring charges, leaving Gokal in career and emotional limbo. His daughter took to social media to bring awareness to the case and set up a GoFundMe fundraising account.[14]

In my native Zambia, people were desperate to have the vaccine as the health-care system was overwhelmed by a second COVID wave, making it the worst surge to occur worldwide at that time. So many things were bungled in its distribution (and it was not done in a socially just way), while in America, some people were refusing what was a precious commodity in short supply in undeveloped countries.

In my family's ancestral home of India, one of the tightest lockdowns worldwide—one that was held up as an example to the rest of the world in many ways—was terminated in October 2020 so schools and businesses, including restaurants, could resume daily operations. Weddings and social events burgeoned. In April 2021, 3.5 million religious devotees gathered in the state of Uttarakhand to participate in the annual holy dip into the sacred Ganges River. Some believed this cleanse would assist in protection from or cure for diseases; others thought it created a spark for India's next wave of COVID-19 infections.

The possibility of a variant strand should also not be negated as potentially contributing to India's catastrophic COVID wave. The delta variant became a household name in the United States and India. Whatever the complex integration of reasons, the healthcare system became completely overwhelmed as people died before they could receive any formal evaluation or treatment. For many, access to the vaccine in India was nearly impossible. Even though 249 million vacations had been given, only a mere 3.4 percent of the country's population was fully vaccinated by June 2021. On May 20, the national daily average death rate peaked at 4,200 deaths. Sadly, many think these numbers were grossly underestimated.

Can you grasp this number? Perhaps most of us know the proverb that one death is a tragedy, while a thousand is a statistic.

Americans, including but not limited to the Appalachian communities discussed earlier as targets of misinformation campaigns, could certainly learn from this situation in India. Appalachia needed to suppress the possibility of yet another COVID wave as schools and businesses returned to regular functions. We needed to remain vigilant and continue to take precautions based on individual circumstances. Politics interfered.

While this pandemic is becoming more controlled, it is still not over. I recall days in 2021 when we were giving up to 300 vaccinations daily in our clinic building, and those setting up appointments

were in tears at the number of people begging to be vaccinated who
had to wait. While our current vaccination numbers are a great
milestone to archive, this country has still suffered the worst hit of
all the nations on earth.

Those who choose not to vaccinate must take extra precautions.
As a doctor, I understand and affirm that choosing not to vaccinate
is a personal decision—but caution patients to examine with care
whose voices they trust, and why, when making that decision. Believing that the entire crisis was manufactured is not tenable. Have
you ever tried to organize a family wedding, planned a conference,
even attempted to pull together a social outing of more than a dozen
people? This worldwide pandemic was not a drill nor a ruse. COVID
has been and, depending on individual and national choices as variants rise, may continue to be, a global crisis. That is all.

### REFERENCES

1 Holshue, M., DeBolt, C., Lindquist, S., et al. First case of 2019 novel
coronavirus in the United States. *New England Journal of Medicine.*
2020;382:929–936. doi:10.1056/NEJMoa2001191.

2 Bodner, J., Welch, W., Brodie, I., Muldoon, A., Leech, D., Marshal,
A. *Covid-19 Conspiracy Theories: QAnon, 5G, the New World Order
and other Viral Ideas.* Jefferson, NC: McFarland; 2021.

3 Harris, T. Grant to study misinformation about the COVID-19 vaccine in Appalachia. Virginia Tech, 2021. https://www.eurekalert.org
/news-releases/490111.

4 Renoud, L., Khouri, C., Revol, B., et al. Association of facial paralysis with mRNA COVID-19 vaccines: a disproportionality analysis using the World Health Organization pharmacovigilance da-
tabase. *JAMA Internal Medicine.* 2021;181(9):1243–1245. doi:10.1001/
jamainternmed.2021.2219.

5 Puente, V. Bridging the great health divide/vaccine divide in Appalachia. WYMT Mountain News, April 1, 2021. https://www.wymt
.com/2021/04/01/bridging-the-great-health-divide-vaccine-divide
-in-appalachia/.

6 Durkee, A. Here are the states with the greatest COVID-19 vaccine hesitancy, poll says. *Forbes,* April 23, 2021. https://www.forbes
.com/sites/alisondurkee/2021/04/23/here-are-the-states-with-the
-greatest-covid-19-vaccine-hesitancy-poll-says/?sh=5f066cf3ead2.

7 Lizarzaburu, J. Forced sterilisation haunts Peruvian women decades on. BBC, December 2, 2015. https://www.bbc.com/news/world-latin-america-34855804.

8 1976: Government admits unauthorized sterilization of Indian women. Native Voices. https://www.nlm.nih.gov/nativevoices/timeline/543.html. Accessed June 16, 2022.

9 Richter, F. COVID-19 has caused a huge amount of lost working hours. World Economic Forum, February 4, 2021. https://www.weforum.org/agenda/2021/02/covid-employment-global-job-loss/.

10 Wang, W. The U.S. divorce rate has hit a 50-year low. Institute for Family Studies, November 10, 2020. https://ifstudies.org/blog/the-us-divorce-rate-has-hit-a-50-year-low.

11 Berger, R. Five breathtaking numbers reveal the unsettling cost of stimulus. Forbes, October 18, 2020. https://www.forbes.com/sites/robertberger/2020/10/18/5-big-numbers-reveal-the-unsettling-scope-of-stimulus-spending/?sh=40c28816142b.

12 Erzurum, S. How much of the population will need to be vaccinated until the pandemic is over? Cleveland Clinic, May 5, 2021. https://health.clevelandclinic.org/how-much-of-the-population-will-need-to-be-vaccinated-until-the-pandemic-is-over/.

13 Wall Street Journal. https://www.wsj.com/livecoverage/covid-2021-05-24. Accessed June 16, 2022.

14 Help Dr. Hasan Gokal to defend himself. GoFundMe. https://www.gofundme.com/f/help-dr-gosan-to-defend-himself. Accessed August 30, 2022.

# 19

## Variants, Vaccines, and Vacations

LAURA HUNGERFORD

*Editor's Note: Delta replaced alpha, and omicron replaced delta. As rates began receding in early 2022, the world held its breath in fear mingled with exhaustion: Was a new variant coming? Ask different questions, Hungerford suggests: When will the next variant arrive, how contagious will it be, and how will it fit into the consideration of COVID as an endemic disease? Most of all, whether another surge appears or not, how do we all use our individual choices to stand for one another against viral invaders, especially when pandemic precautions have been so hard? What will the new normal look like, and will it embrace or ignore the needs of those most at risk?*

As the world began to recognize that a new disease was sweeping across countries and continents in 2020, everyone focused on the virus causing the COVID-19 pandemic: severe acute respiratory syndrome coronavirus-2 (SARS-CoV-2). This virus is in the genus *Betacoronavirus,* which causes the common cold, but members of this genus also produce severe human diseases. Related viruses cause disease in a wide range of animals.[1]

Coronaviruses have a single strand of ribonucleic acid (RNA), which is released into an infected cell and takes over that cell's mechanisms to produce new copies of the virus. We know about the relationships between viruses by studying similarities and differences in these strands of RNA. Larger differences in the RNA genetic code divide viruses into species, but even within the same species, minor variations exist in RNA sequences, producing different strains or variants. This is because small changes continually occur in the genetic code as viruses produce copies of themselves in host cells.

Coronaviruses change more slowly than some other viruses, like human immunodeficiency virus (HIV) or influenza, but more quickly than others, like herpes viruses.[2] A slower mutation rate is good, because it gives people who are infected a chance to develop an immune response that fights that specific variant of the virus, and they are protected for some time after recovery. It also means that people who are vaccinated before they are infected with a particular virus are protected, thereby dramatically decreasing disease and death.

Mutations can occur every time a new copy of a virus is assembled from the basic chemical building blocks. Mutations are just changes in the RNA sequence that happen in several ways. The wrong types of RNA building blocks can be linked, or they can join in the wrong order. Misalignment can occur when subunits of the virus are being attached to each other. Mechanisms in the host cell, trying to thwart viral takeover, can cause lapses in viral construction. SARS-CoV-2 has an internal proofreading enzyme, which works to cut out errors, but some still slip through.[3] Fortunately, most mutations lead to defects that are fatal to the virus, and many others have no effect. Viral mutations can even lead to a virus becoming less dangerous. For example, a widely spreading, mild variant of SARS-CoV-2 could act as a natural vaccine.

But RNA variations can create changes in SARS-CoV-2 that could potentially allow the virus to spread more quickly, cause more severe disease, or evade vaccines or natural immunity. SARS-CoV-2 produces mediators that act within our cells to dampen our immune response, and mutations have already been detected that give variants a greater ability to suppress our defenses within infected cells.[3] Mutations can also occur to change the proteins on the viral surface that are shaped like tiny spikes and bind to specific proteins on host cells as the first step to infection. The SARS-CoV-2 spike protein binds to angiotensin-converting enzyme 2 (ACE2), which is present on cells throughout the body, including in the lungs, nose, mouth and digestive tract, heart, blood vessels, brain, kidney, and liver, and it has an important function to help lower blood pressure and decrease inflammation.[4] A number of other viruses besides SARS-CoV-2 also use ACE2 to enter cells.[3] Mutations have been found within SARS-CoV-2 that allow the spike to bind more quickly or tightly to ACE2, allowing more efficient spread and potentially more severe disease.[5] Current vaccines stimulate an immune response that attacks the spike protein. Boosters or new vaccines may be needed if mutations make a spike that is different enough to evade immunity from vaccination or previous infection.

SARS-CoV-2 viruses that have small changes from the originally sequenced strain have been recognized from very early in the outbreak. Although we did not hear much about variants at first, they have always been there, some spreading, some dying out. The small, continuing RNA changes allow disease detectives to track where coronaviruses are coming from and how they spread. Comparing thousands of samples showed that the first outbreaks were in China, but that an early strain, brought to Europe from China, spread widely, making Europe the source for most subsequent global spread.[6] Similarity between viruses allows public health workers to link cases, improve contact tracing, and help control spread.[7] And when people accidentally infected mink with SARS-CoV-2 (in April 2020 in the Netherlands and later in Denmark, Spain, the United States, and other countries), tracing the small viral mutations showed how the virus was adapting to mink, as well as jumping mink to mink and from mink back to humans.[8] Comparing small genetic changes is already used to fight other diseases. The PulseNet system uses genetic patterns to connect causes of food poisoning across the USA to allow recalls of contaminated vegetables and other foods.[9] Efforts soon began, globally, to track changes in SARS-CoV-2 strains to find and control harmful new variants as early as possible. So far, so good.

The World Health Organization (WHO) has set up a system to track, list, and share information about potentially dangerous variants called "variants of concern" (VOCs).[10] VOCs are those that soon became common in populations, spread more easily or quickly, cause more severe or new types of disease, can't be detected with existing tests, or cause vaccines or treatments to be less effective. These characteristics allowed VOCs to predominate in the second and successive waves of the pandemic (notably in India in mid-2021 and worldwide in late 2021, early 2022, and summer 2022) and raise concerns for any areas or groups that still have low vaccination rates. The US Centers for Disease Control and Prevention (CDC) track VOCs based on their importance within the US.[11] Both the WHO and CDC also track "variants of interest" (VOIs), seen frequently in populations from 2020 on, and have the potential to become VOCs. When VOIs and VOCs become less common and no longer pose a major risk, they are still tracked, but they are reclassified as "variants under monitoring" (VUM) or "variants being monitored" (VBM). When people talk about the threat from SARS-CoV-2 variants, they are generally referring to those on the VOC list.

WHO also proposed a new way to identify the VOI and VOC strains, because the official names are long and somewhat confusing strings of letters and numbers. As a new VOC or VOI is recognized, they are labeled with letters in the Greek alphabet—sort of like hurricanes and typhoons are named each year. The first were labeled as alpha (a.k.a. B.1.1.7 or 201/501Y.V1), beta (a.k.a. B.1.351 or 20H/501. V2), delta (a.k.a. B.1.617.2 or 21A/S:478K), and so on.

By August 2022, the CDC listed one VOC, omicron, noting the multiple worrisome lineages; no current VOIs; and 11 VBMs, including alpha, beta, gamma, and delta, which had previously been listed as VOCs in the United States and internationally. Most of these variants are listed because they seem to spread person to person more quickly or easily. All of them have some reduction in susceptibility to host antibodies, which is not surprising as mutations can change the spike or another viral protein so that it "looks" different to the immune system. So far, none of the variants are able to overwhelm current vaccine or natural immunity.

The chance that a dangerous new variant will emerge is increased by anything that intensifies the numbers of new coronaviruses being produced and breathed or coughed out into the world. So, having more virus replicating in a host, or a longer-lasting infection, or even a mutation that causes faster replication, gives more chances for new strains to emerge and for greater spread to occur. If a sick person spreads infection to one other person, they've just given the virus a fresh, new set of millions of cells to create new viruses and mutations. If the same person completely isolates or the people they contact are vaccinated or wearing masks, they create a dead end for the virus. If they had a mutated virus, that virus dies out. People who forgo vaccination provide a source of new opportunities for mutants to be created and passed on. "Super-spreaders"— that is, one person who spreads SARS-CoV-2 to a whole group or travels and brings the virus to a new place—have played a devastating role in the COVID pandemic.[6,12] It is estimated that 80 percent of COVID cases are spread to others from just 10 percent of all infected individuals, often through contacts in restaurants, group events, or crowded places with poor ventilation. This is especially true in rural areas, where people are more spread out—except when they gather for events.[13] For the delta and omicron variants, transmission from travelers and through social events has led to surges in COVID cases greater than the original wave of this pandemic.[14] Thus, creation and spread of variants isn't just due to the properties of the virus, but also to how we help it along. This gives us an upper hand, if we choose, to slow the spread of mutants.

When we talk about mutations and effects on COVID, it is important to also recognize that human genetic differences affect susceptibility to infection or severe disease. COVID's severity has been linked to the ABO blood type and other genes that we, as humans, have acquired from ancestors from the beginning of time.[15] Variation in the genetic sequence or amount of ACE2 receptor on cells might also affect susceptibility. Gene expression and physiologic changes that occur as people age, between men and women, and among those whose cells are responding to other chronic diseases, for example, may explain why some people are more easily or severely affected by SARS-CoV-2 infections.

Beyond genetic differences, we recognize other factors that increase our risk of disease to SARS-CoV-2 and variants. Older people, men, and those with hypertension, diabetes, and chronic kidney, lung, or heart disease have a higher risk for severe disease and death.[16] For everyone, the more SARS-CoV-2 viruses that you inhale, the more likely you are to be infected and have severe disease, hence the value of wearing masks.[17] In the US, African American / Black and Hispanic populations have higher rates of infection, severe disease, and death. Certain job types, urban areas, housing that leads to more exposure to SARS-CoV-2, as well as less access to health care likely underlie these differences.[18] For rural areas, chronic diseases, aging populations, food insecurity, low levels of access to health care, low vaccination rates, and economic losses create high vulnerability to new outbreaks of COVID.[19] Recognition of these factors has already helped us find ways to protect those at higher risk. With new variants that may spread more quickly or cause more severe disease, individual and collective actions to support health equity will be even more important to keep all parts of our communities safe.

So, what do we do? All viruses rely completely on their host to spread them to a new host. If every person with COVID could immediately and completely isolate themselves, that would be the end of the pandemic. But SARS-CoV-2 is sneaky; it jumps into the air around its infected carriers even before they know that they are infected and can stay in the air in poorly ventilated areas for hours.[20] At least half of the people spreading the virus might never realize that they have it. This means that our measures to stop disease spread need to be implemented by people who seem healthy. Wearing masks, social distancing, being outdoors or in well-ventilated areas, protecting older and vulnerable adults, and not traveling to bring back new variants were very successful in slowing the pandemic.

The addition of extremely effective new vaccines has caused disease, hospitalizations, and deaths to plunge. But public agencies need to monitor SARS-CoV-2 variants, which still threaten us with new waves of disease even as omicron fades. And we each need to be on guard so that we don't pass on a new strain to others. Variants arise and spread whenever we create chances for SARS-CoV-2 to infect and replicate; we must remain proactive to deny this opportunity. We need to be especially careful if we gather with groups of people who are still susceptible to either infection or severe disease. As serious variants could plausibly yet emerge, even those who are vaccinated may need to periodically go back to wearing masks, get additional vaccine boosters, and take other measures. And we must all make sure that we are not the ones who bring along, or bring back, unexpected viral hitchhikers from our vacations as the pandemic becomes endemic.

### REFERENCES

1 Alluwaimi, A.M., Alshubaith, I.H., Al-Ali, A.M., Abohelaika S. The coronaviruses of animals and birds: their zoonosis, vaccines, and models for SARS-CoV and SARS-CoV2. *Frontiers in Veterinary Science.* 2020;7:582287. doi:10.3389/fvets.2020.582287.

2 Duffy, S., Shackelton, L.A., Holmes, E.C. Rates of evolutionary change in viruses: patterns and determinants. *Nature Reviews Genetics.* 2008;9(4):267–276. doi:10.1038/nrg2323.

3 Christie, M.J., Irving, A.T., Forster, S.C., et al. Of bats and men: immunomodulatory treatment options for COVID-19 guided by the immunopathology of SARS-CoV-2 infection. *Science Immunology.* 2021;6(63):eabd0205. doi:10.1126/sciimmunol.abd0205.

4 Perrotta, F., Matera, M.G., Cazzola, M., Bianco, A. Severe respiratory SARS-CoV2 infection: does ACE2 receptor matter? *Respiratory Medicine.* 2020;168:105996. doi:10.1016/j.rmed.2020.105996.

5 Lauring, A.S., Hodcroft, E.B. Genetic variants of SARS-CoV-2—what do they mean? *JAMA.* 2021;325(6):529–531. doi:10.1001/jama.2020.27124.

6 Rito, T., Richards, M.B., Pala, M., Correia-Neves, M., Soares, P.A. Phylogeography of 27,000 SARS-CoV-2 genomes: Europe as the major source of the COVID-19 pandemic. *Microorganisms.* 2020;8(11):1678–1691. doi:10.3390/microorganisms8111678.

7 Pfefferle, S., Günther, T., Kobbe, R., et al. SARS Coronavirus-2 variant tracing within the first Coronavirus Disease 19 clusters in north-

ern Germany. *Clinical Microbiology and Infection.* 2021;27(1):130. e5–130.e8. doi:10.1016/j.cmi.2020.09.034.

8  Mallapaty S. COVID mink analysis shows mutations are not dangerous—yet. *Nature.* 2020;587(7834):340–341. doi:10.1038/d41586 -020-03218-z.

9  Marshall, K.E., Nguyen, T.A., Ablan, M., et al. Investigations of possible multistate outbreaks of *Salmonella,* shiga toxin-producing *Escherichia coli,* and *Listeria monocytogenes* infections—United States. *MMWR Surveillance Summaries.* 2016;69(6):1–14. doi:10.15585/mmwr.ss6906a1.

10 Tracking SARS-CoV-2 variants. World Health Organization, December 31, 2021. https://www.who.int/en/activities/tracking-SARS -CoV-2-variants.

11 SARS-CoV-2 variant classifications and definitions. Centers for Disease Control, December 1, 2021 (updated April 26, 2022). https:// www.cdc.gov/coronavirus/2019-ncov/variants/variant-info.html.

12 Lewis, D. The superspreading problem. *Nature.* 2021;590:544–546. https://media.nature.com/original/magazine-assets/d41586-021 -00460-x/d41586-021-00460-x.pdf.

13 Lau, M.S.Y., Grenfell, B., Thomas, M., Bryan, M., Nelson, K., Lopman, B. Characterizing superspreading events and age-specific infectiousness of SARS-CoV-2 transmission in Georgia, USA. *Proceedings of the National Academy of Sciences.* 2020;117(36):22430–22435. doi:10.1073/pnas.2011802117.

14 Espenhain, L., Funk, T., Overvad, M., et al. Epidemiological characterisation of the first 785 SARS-CoV-2 Omicron variant cases in Denmark, December 2021. *Eurosurveillance.* 2021;26(50):2101146. doi:10.2807/1560-7917.ES.2021.26.50.2101146.

15 Zeberg, H., Pääbo, S. The major genetic risk factor for severe COVID-19 is inherited from Neanderthals. *Nature.* 2020;587:610–612. doi:10.1038/s41586-020-2818-3.

16 Li, J., Huang, D.Q., Zou B., et al. Epidemiology of COVID-19: a systematic review and meta-analysis of clinical characteristics, risk factors, and outcomes. *Journal of Medical Virology.* 2021;93(3):1449–1458. doi:10.1002/jmv.26424.

17 Spinelli, M.A., Glidden, D.V., Gennatas, E.D., et al. Importance of non-pharmaceutical interventions in lowering the viral inoculum to reduce susceptibility to infection by SARS-CoV-2 and potentially disease severity. *Lancet Infectious Diseases.* 2021;21(9):E296–E301. doi:10.1016/S1473-3099(20)30982-8.

18 Mackey, K., Ayers, C.K., Kondo, K.K., et al. Racial and ethnic disparities in COVID-19-related infections, hospitalizations, and deaths: a

systematic review. *Annals of Internal Medicine.* 2021;174(3):362–373. doi:10.7326/M20-6306.

19 Henning-Smith, C. The unique impact of COVID-19 on older adults in rural areas. *Journal of Aging & Social Policy.* 2020;32(4–5):396–402. doi:10.1080/08959420.2020.1770036.

20 Tang, J.W., Marr, L.C., Li, Y., Dancer, S.J. COVID-19 has redefined airborne transmission. *BMJ.* 2021;373:n913. doi:10.1136/bmj.n913.

# Contributors

LUCAS AIDUKAITIS graduated from the Dr. S. Hughes Melton Family Medicine Residency Program at Johnston Memorial Hospital. He lives with his wife and their five children in Abingdon, Virginia, but hails from the southern state of Rio Grande do Sul, Brazil.

CLAY ANDERSON holds an undergraduate degree in biological sciences from the University of South Carolina, a master's degree in behavioral neuroscience from Georgia State University, and a medical doctorate from the Medical University of South Carolina. After residency, he plans to practice in South Carolina.

TAMMY BANNISTER, a lifelong resident of West Virginia and a coal miner's daughter, grew up to be a family physician and practice in her Appalachian home. She is currently professor and program director for the Marshall Family Medicine Residency in Huntington, West Virginia.

ALLI DELP grew up in a small town and decided to become a doctor after her brother was diagnosed with cancer. Mother, wife, daughter, sister, aunt, and friend, she is also assistant director in a Family Medicine Residency, where she teaches future doctors the joys of big lives in small towns.

LYNN ELLIOTT has lived in Abingdon, Virginia, for nine years. She has held positions in academic administration at Memorial Sloan-Kettering Cancer Center and later served as registrar and residency coordinator at the UCLA School of Medicine. She holds a master of divinity from Princeton Theological Seminary.

MONIKA HOLBEIN is a palliative care and hospice physician at Penn State Health. She has a special interest in treating patients with cancer and walking with them on their cancer journey. She enjoys spending time with her family in the great outdoors.

LAURA HUNGERFORD is an infectious disease epidemiologist and heads Virginia Tech's Public Health Program and the Population Health Sciences Department in the Virginia-Maryland College of Veterinary Medicine. Her research includes collaborative studies that take a One Health approach to infectious diseases, GIS and spatial statistical analyses, and dynamic modeling involving raccoons, frogs, birds, aquatic animals, and other species.

NIKKI KING is a native of Kentucky and earned her doctorate in health-care administration at the Medical University of South Carolina in 2021.

JEFFREY LEBOEUF, CAE, grew up in rural south Louisiana. He received an MBA and a master's of health administration from the University of Missouri after completing undergraduate work in business administration from Louisiana State University. Currently pursuing a doctorate in higher education administration, he has been involved in osteopathic medical administration since 1997 and in graduate medical education leadership since 2009.

SOJOURNER NIGHTINGALE is the pseudonym of a nurse in rural Appalachia. She became a nurse after watching family members die from illnesses that were not fatal among White neighbors. When not nursing, she is raising a family on a farm.

BETH O'CONNOR has lived in rural communities her entire life, except while earning her master's degree at the University of Cincinnati. Executive director of Virginia Rural Health Association since 2005, she was elected National Rural Health Association president for 2022. A dedicated advocate, she started her first petition at age 14.

RAKESH PATEL is a native of Zambia and moved to Texas at 16 and obtained a bachelor's degree in respiratory therapy, followed by a medical degree and master of business administration. After completing his residency in internal medicine at Johnston Memorial Hospital, he plans to pursue a fellowship in pulmonology / critical care.

MILDRED F. PERREAULT is an assistant professor in the Department of Media and Communication at East Tennessee State University. Perreault's research program seeks to understand the role of mediated communication in crises and natural disasters. Her work has been published in *American Behavioral Scientist, Disasters, Health Communication,* and *Traumatology.*

MELANIE B. RICHARDS is an associate professor in the Department of Media and Communication at East Tennessee State University. Richards previously served in leadership roles for the American Cancer Society and Teach for America. Her research focuses on nonprofit and health communication and the scholarship of teaching and learning.

TARA SMITH is an internal medicine physician who earned her medical degree from Lincoln Memorial University in Harrogate, Tennessee, near her home town of Pineville, Kentucky. She practices in Lexington.

KATHY OSBORNE STILL retired as communication director for UVA Wise in 2021. She also served as UVA Wise spokesperson, freedom of information officer, and editor of the *UVA Wise Magazine.* She chaired the college's crisis communication team and was an award-winning reporter for the *Bristol Herald Courier.*

DARLA TIMBO, PsyD, LPC, has 13-plus years in the field of psychology and counseling. An assistant professor in the Department of Criminal Justice and Psychology at California University of Pennsylvania, she teaches in the undergraduate psychology program. Her current research includes multiculturalism and client outcomes in therapy.

WENDY WELCH, director of the Southwest Virginia Graduate Medical Education Consortium, is the author of *The Little Bookstore of Big Stone Gap* and *Fall or Fly: The Strangely Hopeful Story of Adoption and Foster Care in Appalachia;* coauthor of *COVID-19*

*Conspiracy Theories: QAnon, 5G, the New World Order and Other Viral Ideas;* and editor of *From the Front Lines of the Appalachian Addiction Crisis* and *Public Health in Appalachia.* Her blog is found at wendy-welch.com. She is researching medical mistrust, housing stability, and food insecurity tie-ins.

KATHY WIBBERLY is director of the Mid-Atlantic Telehealth Resource Center, director of research for the Karen S. Rheuban Center for Telehealth, and assistant professor of public health sciences at the University of Virginia School of Medicine. Kathy's public health career of 30-plus years has focused on policy, program development/ evaluation, and strategic planning.

# Index

trauma (*cont.*)
  societal, based on racism, 202,
  217. *See also under* Black people
  trust, 78, 149, 151, 201, 203, 206,
  210, 221, 268, 279

US Department of Health and
  Human Services (DHHS), 17,
  53, 58, 264

vaccination, non-COVID, 20, 29,
  276
VAERS (Vaccine Adverse Event
  Reporting System), 209

WHO (World Health Organization), 267, 285